Animal Kingdom presents

Power Isotonics

The Complete Book of Dynamic Self-Resistance Exercises for Men and Women

By David Nordmark

www.animal-kingdom-workouts.com

Disclaimer

The exercises and advice contained within this course may be too strenuous or dangerous for some people, and the reader(s) should consult a physician before engaging in them.

The author and publisher of this course are not responsible in any manner whatsoever for any injury which may occur through reading and following the instructions herein.

Power Isotonics - The Complete Book of Dynamic Self-Resistance Exercises for Men and Women

No part of this course may be reproduced or transmitted in any form or by any means, electronic or mechanical, including photocopying, recording, or by any information storage and retrieval system, without permission in writing from the publisher.

Copyright © 2010 David Nordmark. All rights reserved.
www.Animal-Kingdom-Workouts.com

Table of Contents

Introduction — *6*
How To Perform These Exercises — 7
Some Notes On Diet — 8

Workout Routines — *9*
Beginner Workout Routine — 9
Advanced Workout Routine — 10

Chest Exercises — *11*
Deep Breathing Chest Expander — 13
Deep Breathing Chest Flex — 15
Atlas Pushups — 17
Chest Builder — 19
Rope Pull — 21
Chest Crosses — 23
Pectoral Presses — 25
Chest Presses — 27
Chest Squeeze — 29

Abdominal Exercises — *31*
Isometric Stomach Flattener — 33
The Iso-Vacuum — 35
Leg Raise — 37
Concentrated Sit-Ups — 39
Leg Cross Raises — 41
Side Bends — 43

Torso Twisting	45

Exercises For The Neck — **47**

Front Neck Conditioner	49
Rear Neck Conditioner	51
Side Neck Conditioner	53
Side Neck Twist	55
Neck Rotations	57

Shoulder Exercises — **59**

Shoulder Pushes	61
Elbow Presses	63
Shoulder Shrugs	65
Shoulder Extensions	67
Shoulder Pulls	69
Shoulder Raises	71
Shoulder Rotations	73

Exercises For The Back And Spine — **75**

Sitting Spine Twist	77
Upper Spine Stretch	79
Standing Spine Twist	81
Standing Spine Bends	83
Spine Spirals	85
Isotonic Deadlift	87
Sitting Back Pull	89
Shoulder Blade Contraction	91
Back Flex	93

Standing Back Flex	95
Arm Exercises	**97**
Biceps Curls	99
Triceps Press Down	101
Arm Rotations	103
Concentration Curls	105
Concentration Flexes	107
Leg Exercises	**109**
Frog Squats	111
Sitting Leg Flexes	113
Sitting Leg Extensions	115
Leg Curls	117
Thigh Flexes	119
Leg Kicks	121
Calve Press Ups	123
Other Courses	**125**

Introduction

Joe Lois did them. So did Joe Dimaggio. Charles Atlas, "The Worlds Most Perfectly Developed Man", put out a famous mail order course on them (although he called them Dynamic Tension). What are they? Isotonic Exercises. This proven form of exercise will allow you to burn fat, build muscle and sculpt your body in record time. What's more all this can be done anywhere at anytime and requires no special weights, gym or equipment. How is this possible? Because the Power Isotonic exercises that follow make use of your own body and bodyweight. That's right, your body is the gym. Let me explain.

Strictly defined, an isotonic exercise is a form of exercise which involves controlled contraction and extension of the muscles and mobilization of the joints around those muscles. For an exercise to be isotonic the joints do move and the muscles do elongate (or contract) but the tension causing this remains the same. What this means is that an exercise like weight lifting is in fact an isotonic exercise. Weightlifting, however, is the road most commonly travelled. You can build muscle this way, but it's not the only way. It may not even be the best way.

Power Isotonics is the other, less well travelled path to optimum physical fitness. With the exercises that follow you will either be using your own bodyweight or making use of self-resistance (pitting one limb against the other) in order to achieve the same effect. However there are three big advantages to this form of training over traditional weightlifting. They are:

Safety - Power Isotonics is much safer than weightlifting. The reason for this is that one's own muscles provide the resistance. It's almost impossible to overtrain due to the fact that when your muscles tire the resistance will naturally decrease as well. I've known of bodybuilders who have torn there pectoral muscles clear from the bone in an effort to build a powerful chest. This is literally impossible with Power Isotonics.

Convenience - Because your body is your gym, you can literally work out anywhere at anytime. I've known some people (myself included) who will take a break from the computer and do a few Power Isotonic exercises throughout the day. Not only does this help keep you alert during the day (and it's much healthier than grabbing a cup of coffee) but it saves you time as well.

Effectiveness - So long as you concentrate and put all of your energies into them, these exercises are incredibly effective. One of the main reasons for this is related to why they are so safe in the first place. On the one hand when you get tired, the force you are using will naturally decrease. On the other hand as you get stronger, the exercises will naturally become more intense. You will never have to guess exactly how much weight to use to progress. Your body will do this naturally.

The last point begs the question, however. If exercises like Power Isotonics are so effective and were in fact used by athletes as diverse as Joe Dimaggio and Joe Louis in the past, why aren't they in great use today? There are many reasons for this but I suspect the big reason is commerce. The weight loss and fitness industries are huge. It is largely based on selling people all kinds of equipment and supplements with the hope of getting fit. What do you think would happen to this industry if people got the word that they didn't need expensive gym memberships or diet pills? I think the answer is fairly obvious.

How To Perform These Exercises

When performing any of the Power Isotonic exercises there are two things you really need to focus on in order to gain maximum benefits. These are your breath and your mind.

The breath is important because in order to develop your muscles fully it is vitally important that they be continually supplied with fresh oxygen. Inhaling deeply and fully is how you accomplish this. Think of it this way. Your lungs are almost triangle shape, narrow at the top and wide at the bottom. When you take in a shallow breath you are only filling up the top of your lungs. This means your blood is only getting a small percentage of the fresh air that it could be getting. This is why it is so important to always breath deeply from your diaphragm. Unless otherwise noted, alway take in a deep breath of air at the start of a repetition as this will ensure you get the maximum oxygen to your lungs which will result in maximum muscle growth.

Your mind is the second item you must learn to use effectively in order to get the maximum benefit from this course. When you perform the Power Isotonic exercises really picture in your minds eye which muscles you are working and how you want them to look. Don't let your mind wander thinking about the bills you need to pay or the groceries you need to buy. Always remember that you brain commands your muscles. When your mind is focused your muscles will respond much more quickly.

Some Notes On Diet

To legendary fitness pioneer Jack Lalanne, exercise was the King of a healthy body but proper diet was the Queen. If you want to be in the truly best shape you can be it is important to eat a clean diet as often as possible. This means that you will want to strive to eat food in as close to its natural state as possible. The more you avoid the overly processed food that you typically find in bags, boxes or wrappers the better.

Workout Routines

Now that you've read all of the above you are getting very close to the actual exercises themselves. Where do you begin? The first thing you need to understand is that due to the intense nature of these exercises each exercise needs to be performed with a days rest in between in order to get the maximum benefits. The reason for this is that when you perform intense exercise you are actually breaking down individual muscle cells. Once you have done this your body starts to repair these cells by pumping in nutrient rich blood. The muscles then heal except bigger and stronger than before. This is also why nutrition is so important when following a fitness program. Your body needs healthy food to grow.

Beginner Workout Routine

When you are just starting out I suggest you perform all of the chest exercises, starting with the two deep breathing ones, for 1 week. As you are always resting between exercises for a day this would mean performing them 3 to 4 times in the course of a week. The reason you are starting with the chest exercises is that they are the best at training your body to accept large amounts of oxygen. This energizes your body and will prepare you for the coming weeks.

Once you have done the chest exercises for at least a week it is time to start adding in additional exercises. While still performing all of the chest exercises I suggest you pick one or two exercises from each of the remaining sections to add to your routine. So from the Abdominal Exercises section you might pick the Isometric Stomach Flattener. From the Shoulder Exercises section you might pick Shoulder Pushes, and so on. Perform the exercises in this fashion, changing the exercises as you like, for another 2 weeks minimum.

At this point your body should be used to working out and you can start to focus on areas in which you really want to see rapid improvement. Let's say you really want larger arms with greater definition. In this case, you would perform a breathing exercise followed by one of the chest exercises (instead of doing all of them), one or two exercises from the rest of the sections, and then finish off with ALL of the arm exercises. Do this 3 or 4 times, always resting for a day between workouts, for at least a week. Once the week is up you can either keep working on your arms or change things up and focus on another body part.

To Summarize, this is the beginning workout routine I would recommend.

- Week 1
    - All chest exercises
- Week 2,3
    - All chest exercises while adding one or two exercises from the other sections
- Week 4
    - Begin with a deep breathing exercise (like the Deep Breathing Chest Expander). Now perform a one or two exercises from the other sections, plus all from one area you want to focus on. Do this for at least a week and then change it up as you wish.

Advanced Workout Routine

You will see great results if you simply perform the beginning workout routine 3 or 4 times a week. If you wish to take it to another level, however you can start to train six days a week (I suggest resting on the 7th). How do you do this while still resting for a day between exercises? Simple. All you need to do is to break up the exercises. So, on Monday, Wednesday, Friday you might perform all of the upper body exercises. On Tuesday, Thursday, Saturday you perform the lower body exercises. Performing Power Isotonics this way allows you to utilize all of the exercises while still getting the required rest.

Chest Exercises

It's a good idea to start your isotonic exercises with some chest exercises. The reason for this is that they bring in a lot of extra oxygen into the body which will energize you for the workout to follow. Aside from that the purpose of the pectoral muscles is to move the arms downwards, forwards, and across the chest. These muscles greatly enhance one's physique and can greatly aid one's ability in all racquet and combat sports.

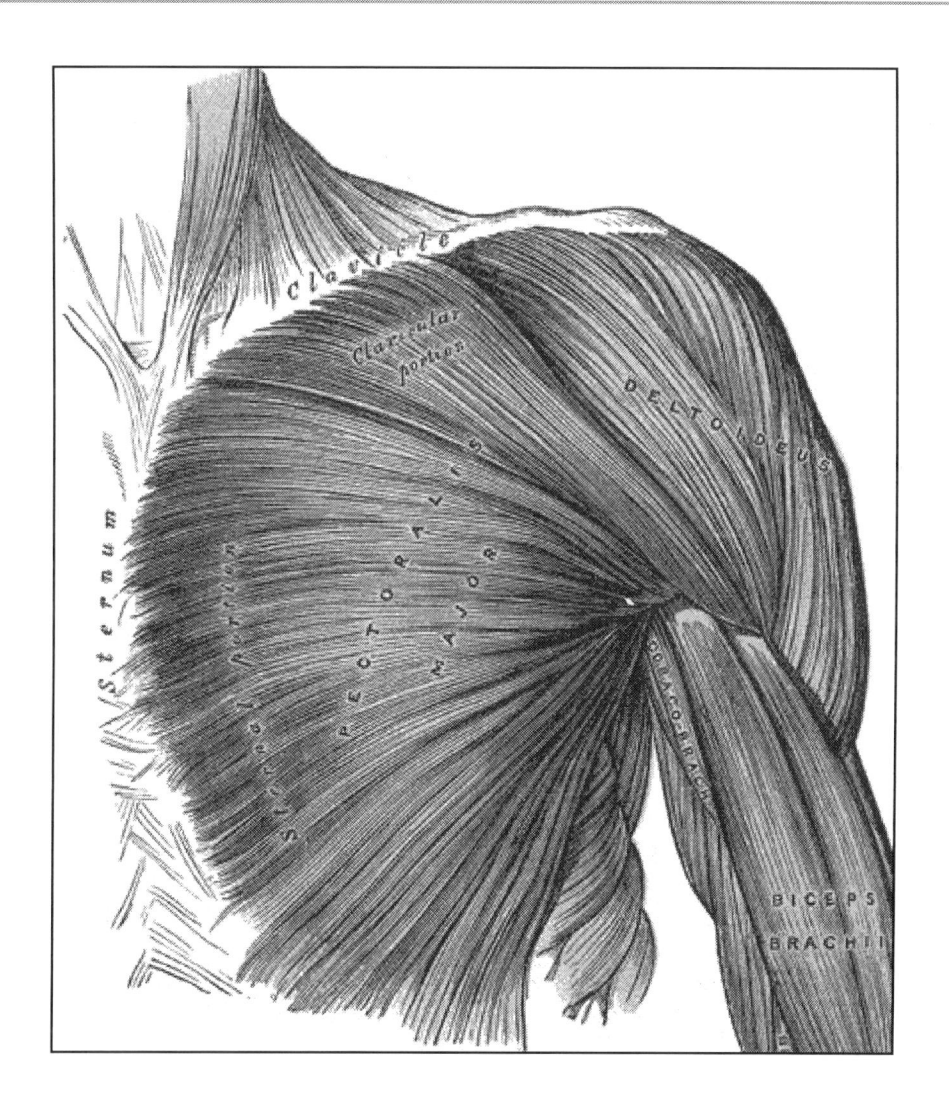

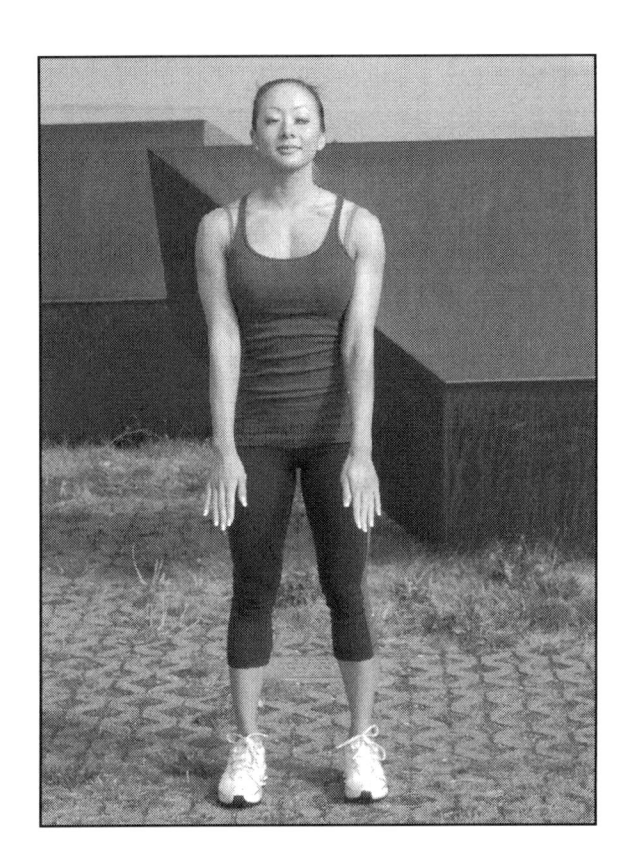

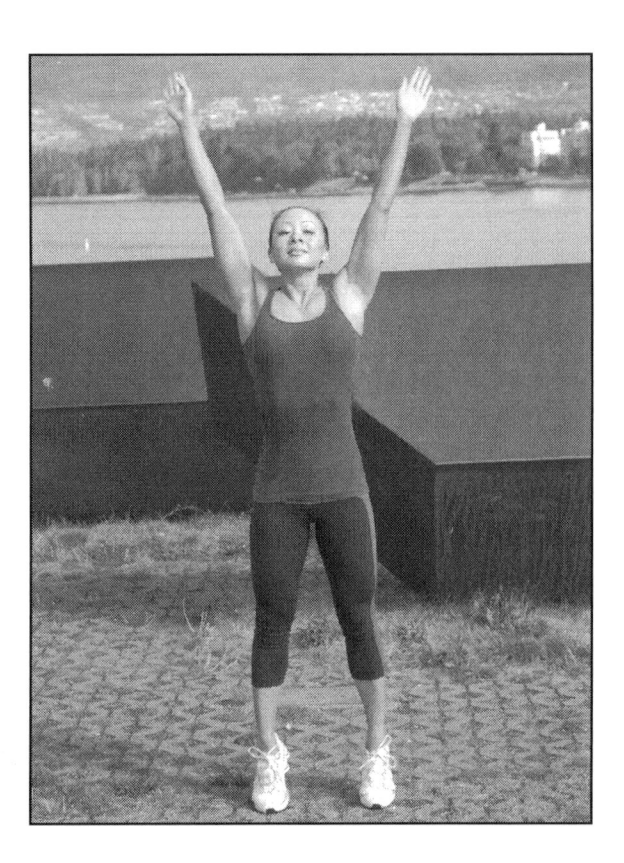

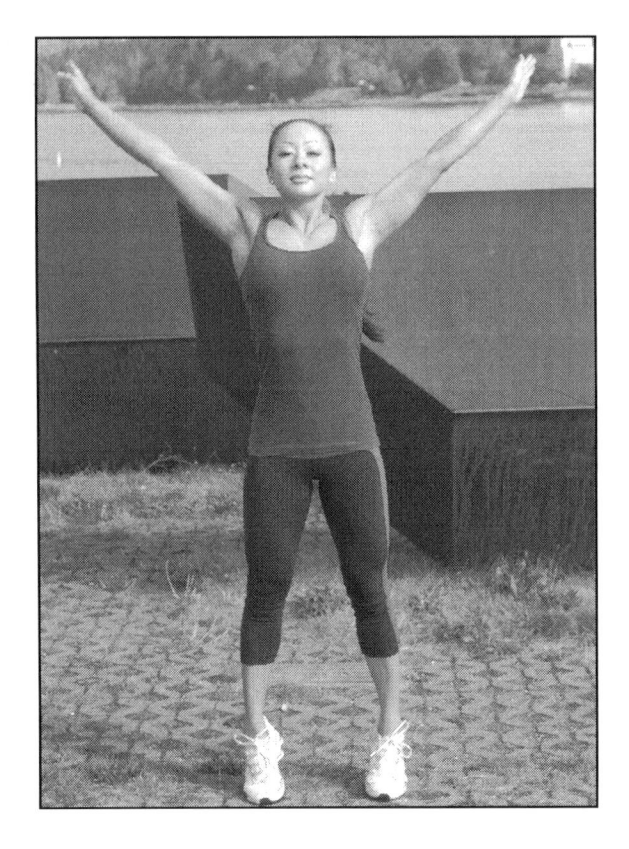

Copyright © 2010 David Nordmark. All rights reserved.
www.animal-kingdom-workouts.com

Page 12

Deep Breathing Chest Expander

This is the one exercise that should be done everyday. If possible, try and perform it outside or by an open window in order to breathe in fresh air. This exercise will get the oxygen flowing through your body while expanding your rib cage and adding to the size of your chest.

Number Of Repetitions

Beginner: 10 repetitions

Intermediate: 20 repetitions

Advanced: 30 repetitions

How To Perform The Exercise

1. Stand with your feet shoulder width apart and your hands by your sides.
2. Breathe in through your nose as you perform the following in one motion. Rise up on your toes while you raise your arms straight out in front of you and then up and out to the sides.
3. Exhale as you lower you hands to your side.
4. You should now be back in the starting position with your feet flat on the floor.

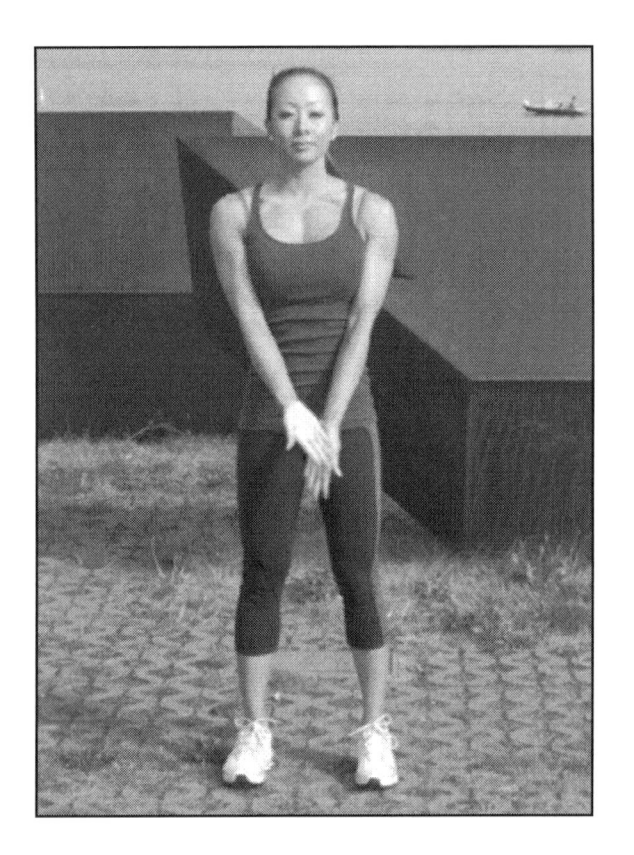

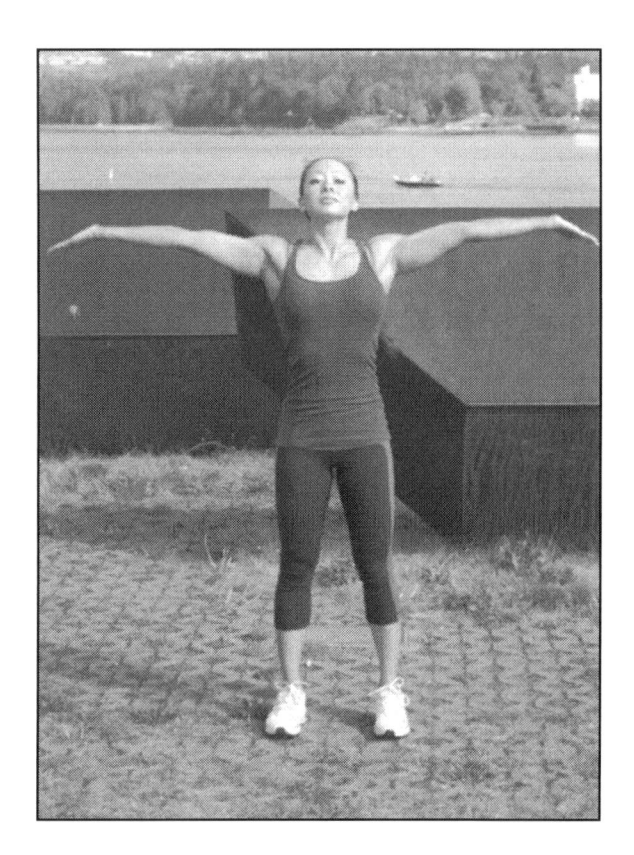

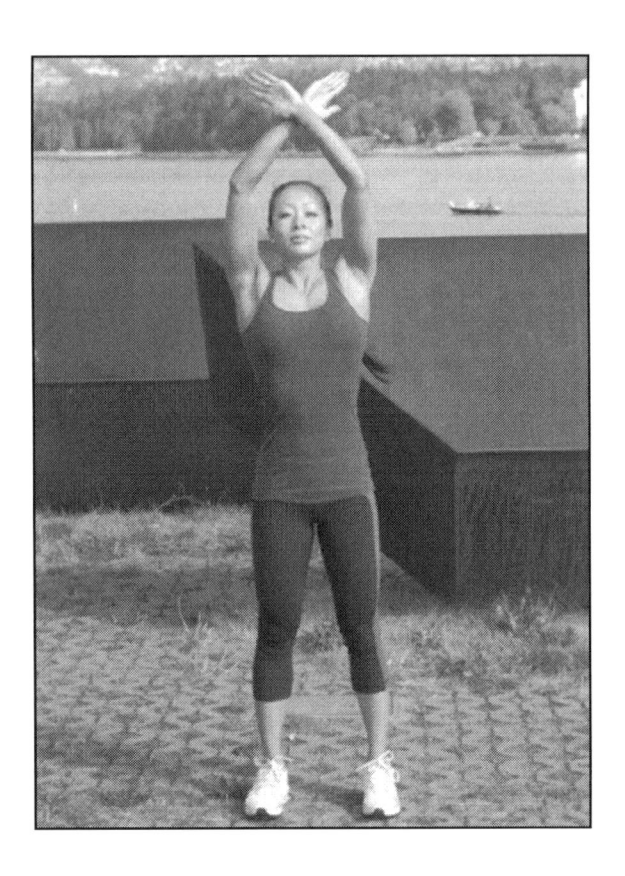

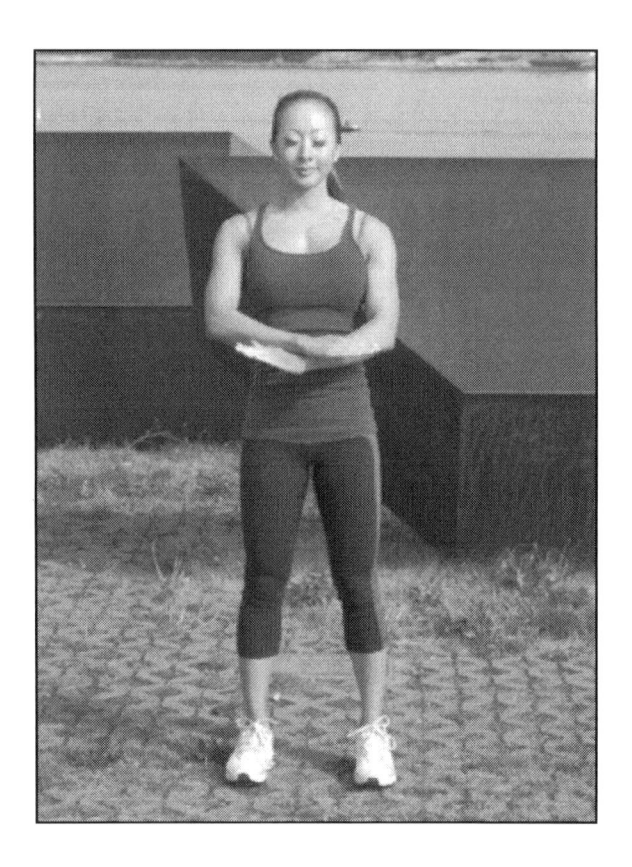

Copyright © 2010 David Nordmark. All rights reserved.
www.animal-kingdom-workouts.com

Deep Breathing Chest Flex

This is another deep breathing exercise that will help you build a powerful chest.

Number Of Repetitions

Beginner: 15 repetitions

Intermediate: 30 repetitions

Advanced: 60 repetitions

How To Perform The Exercise

1. Begin with your feet shoulder width apart and your arms by your sides.
2. Keeping your arms straight, raise your arms in a circular motion till they are above your head.
3. Really stretch your arms to the sides so that your feel it in your arms, shoulders and lats.
4. When your arms reach the top of your head cross your arms at the wrists and bring them down straight in front of your chest.
5. During this downwards motion make sure you flex your chest muscles.
6. Inhale through your nose as you raise your arms and exhale during the downwards motion.

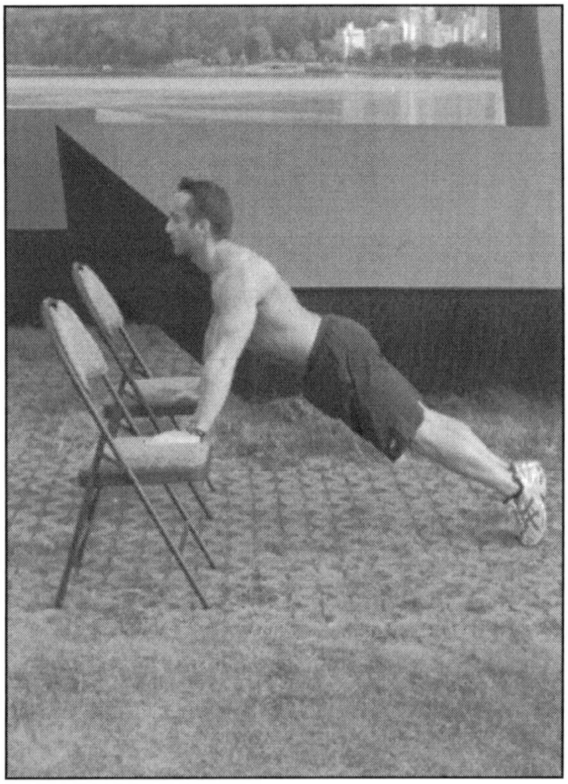

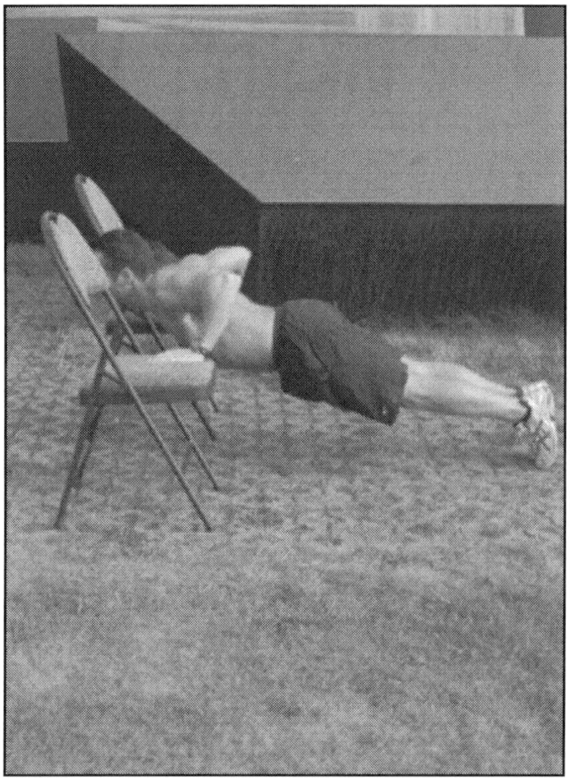

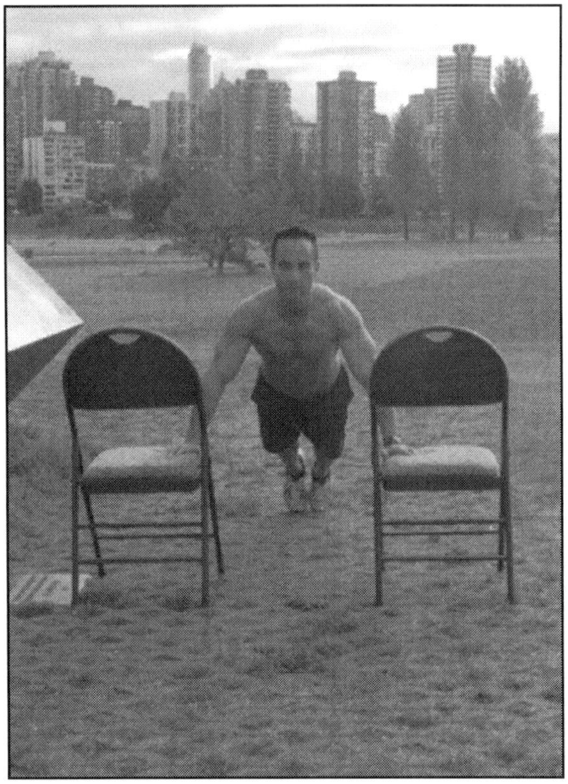

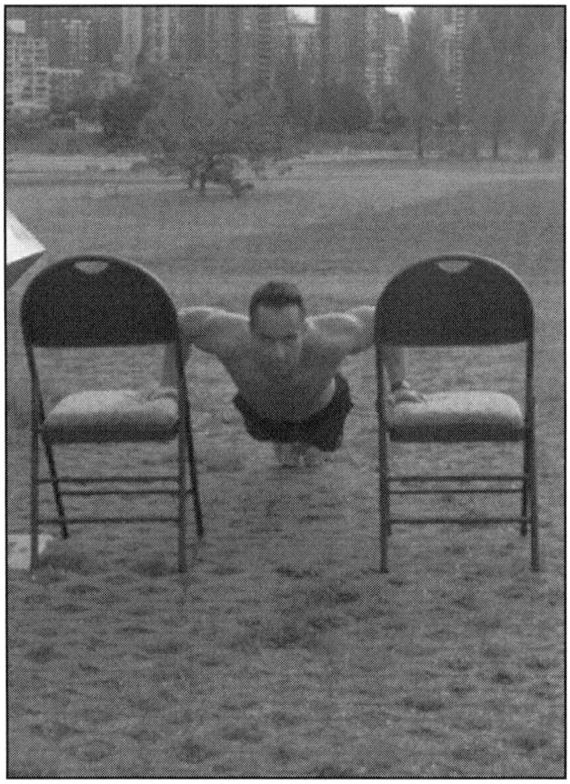

Atlas Pushups

Atlas Pushups are a form of pushup popularized by the legendary Charles Atlas. In order to perform them you will need two sturdy chairs. This exercise really works the chest, arms, and back.

Number Of Repetitions

Beginner: 20 repetitions

Intermediate: 40 repetitions

Advanced: 100 repetitions

How To Perform The Exercise

1. Place two chairs side by side about 18 inches apart.
2. Place each of your hands on the seat of the chairs with your arms straight. The rest of your body should be straight as well with it extended to the floor. This is the starting position.
3. Bend your elbows and lower yourself between the chairs as far as you can go.
4. Push yourself back up to the starting position. Breathe in as you lower yourself, breathe out as you push yourself back up.

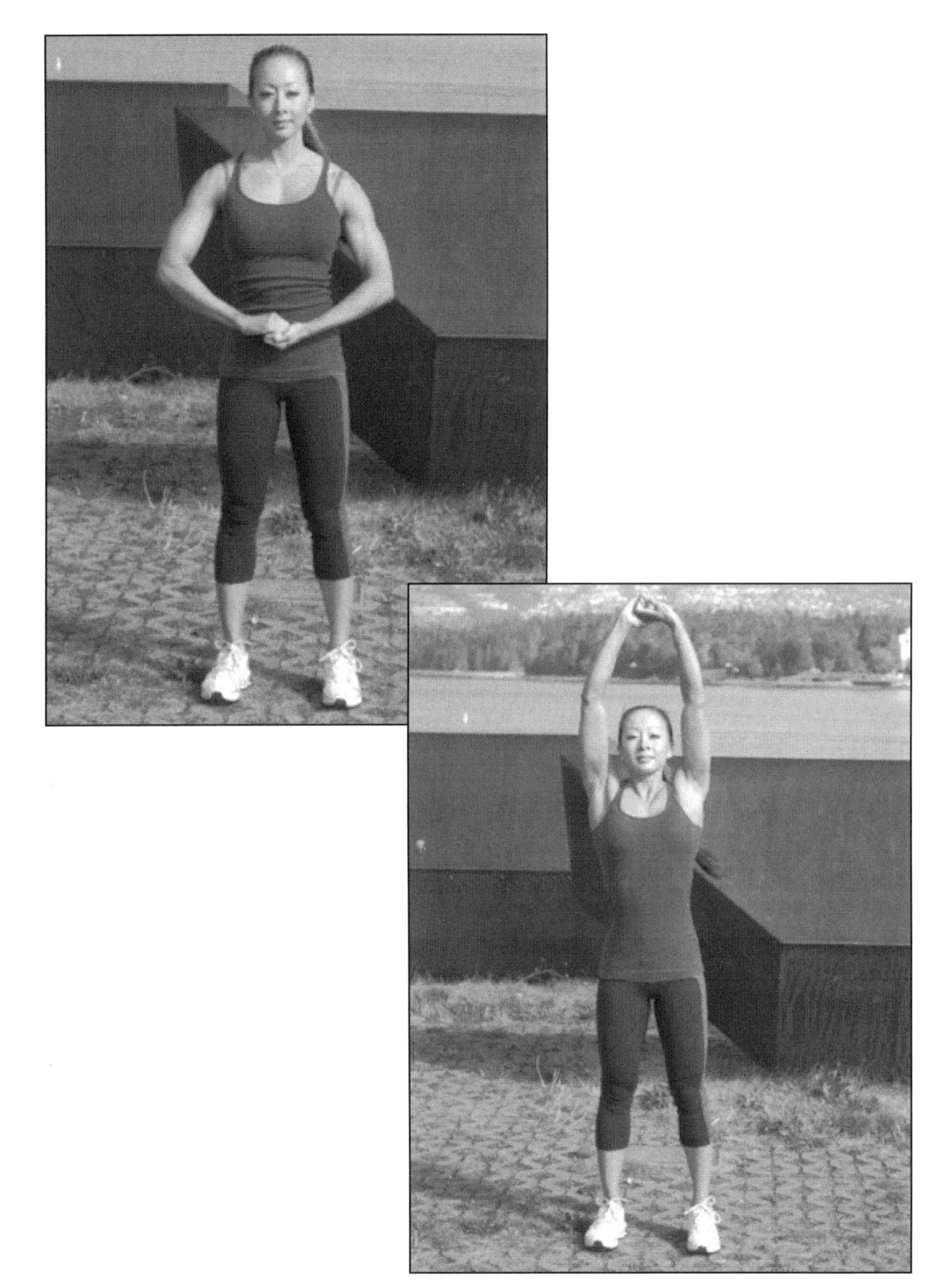

Chest Builder

This exercise will help you build strength as well as definition in your chest.

Number Of Repetitions

Beginner: 20 repetitions

Intermediate: 30 repetitions

Advanced: 40 repetitions

How To Perform The Exercise

1. Begin with your feet shoulder width apart and your fingers clasped in front of you at your waist.
2. Clasp your hands so that your left palm's is facing upwards and your right is facing the floor.
3. Keeping your hands firmly clasped use your chest and arm muscles in order to try and separate your hands. As you do so, raise your hands above your head and then lower them again to your waist level.
4. Inhale through your nose as you raise your hands, exhale as you lower them.
5. When your hands return to waist level release the tension by reversing the hand grip.

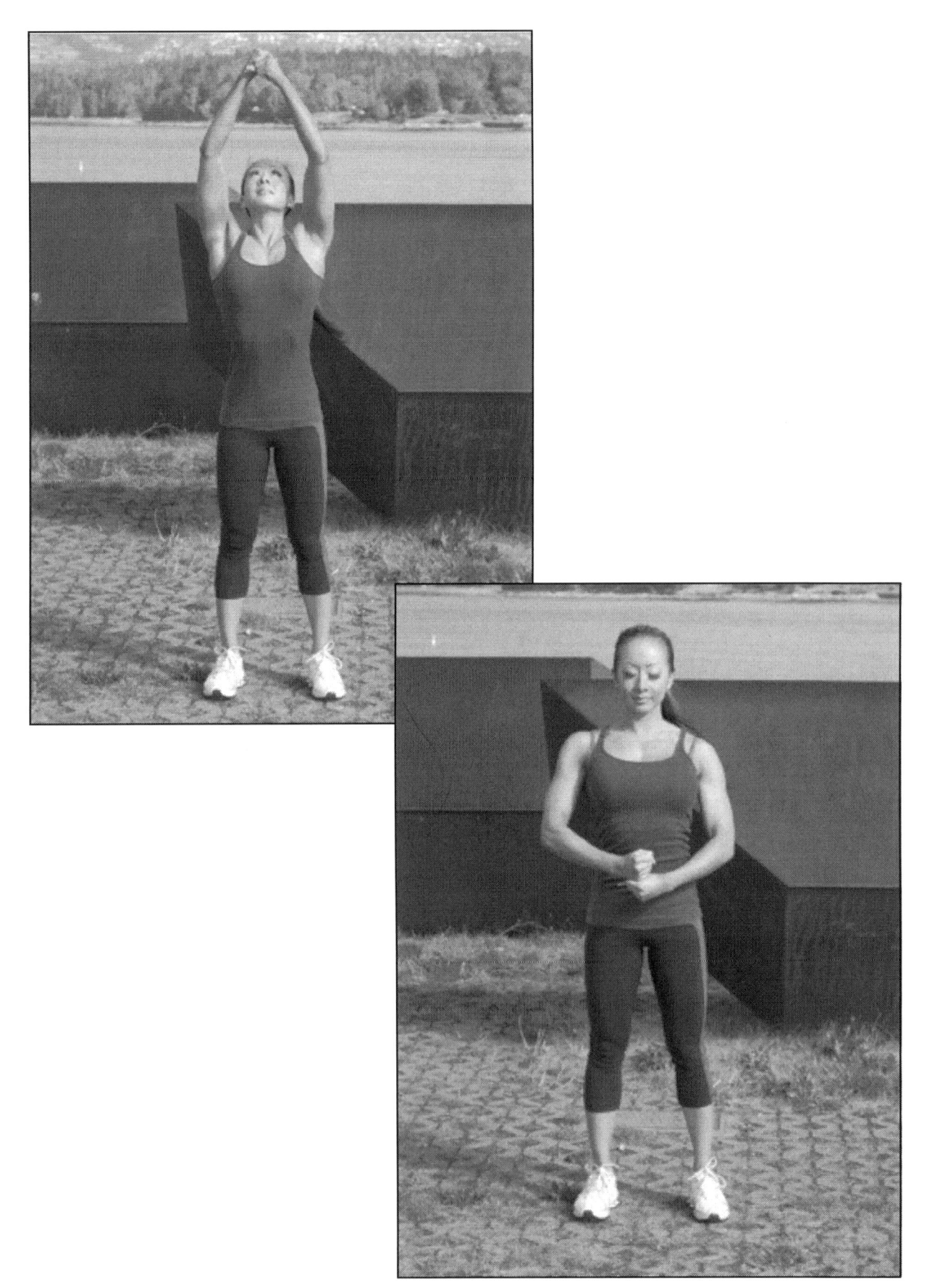

Rope Pull

This exercise will help you build strength as well as definition in your chest.

Number Of Repetitions

Beginner: 10 repetitions

Intermediate: 20 repetitions

Advanced: 40 repetitions

How To Perform The Exercise

1. With your feet shoulder width apart and knees slightly bent put your hands into fists.
2. Raise your arms so that your fists are above your head. Place one of your fists on top of the other, almost like you're grabbing an imaginary rope.
3. Flex your chest muscles as your lower your fists to waist level.
4. As your lower your fists create some additional tension by resisting the downwards motion of the upper fist with the one on the bottom.
5. Inhale when your raise your arms above your head, exhale as your lower them.
6. Make sure you alternate which fist is in the top position so that you develop your muscles evenly.

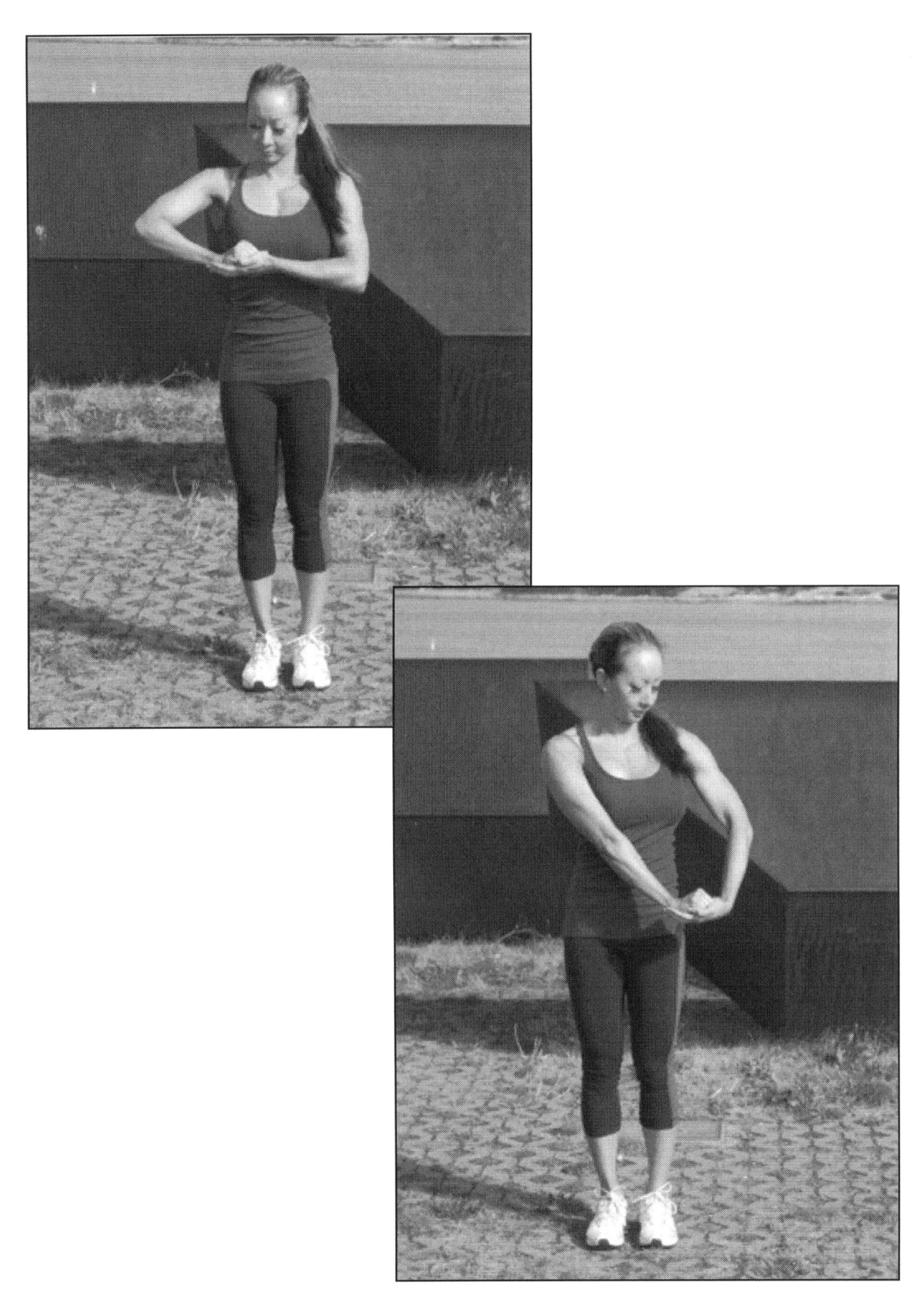

Copyright © 2010 David Nordmark. All rights reserved.
www.animal-kingdom-workouts.com

Page 22

Chest Crosses

Number Of Repetitions

Beginner: 10 (5 per side) repetitions

Intermediate: 20 (10 per side) repetitions

Advanced: 40 (20 per side) repetitions

How To Perform The Exercise

1. Begin with your arms relaxed by your sides and your feet shoulder width apart.
2. Bend your right arm 90 degrees at the elbow and so that your open right palm is facing upwards at chest level.
3. Make a fist with your left hand and place it into your right palm. This is the starting position.
4. Resisting with your right arm press your left fist downwards and towards the right side. At the end of the motion your left arm should almost be straight and diagonal against your body.
5. Repeat this motion with the arms reversed.
6. Inhale through your nose as you get your arms into the starting position. Exhale as you press your arms downwards.

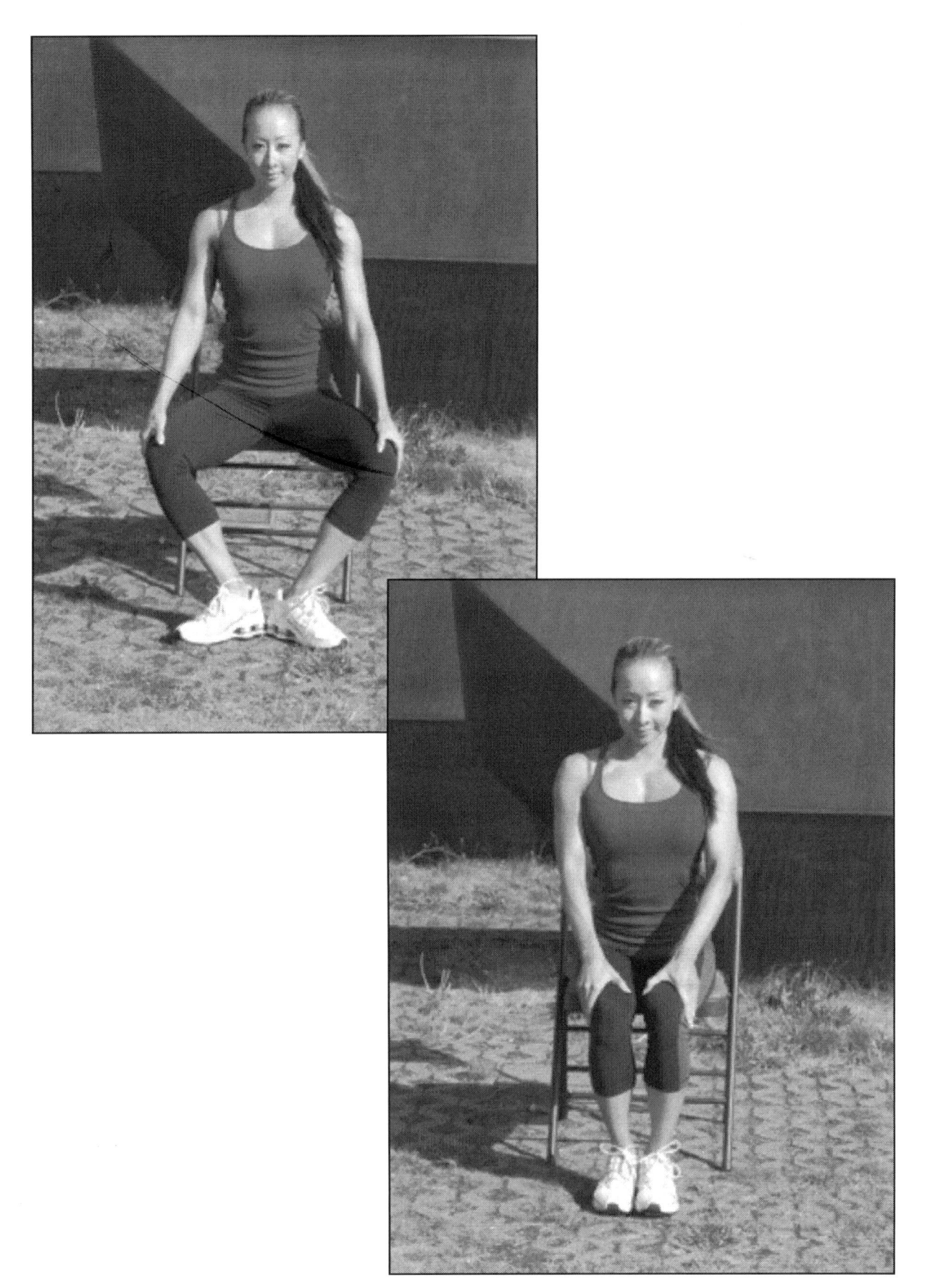

Copyright © 2010 David Nordmark. All rights reserved.
www.animal-kingdom-workouts.com

Page 24

Pectoral Presses

This exercise will help you build your pectoral muscles which will give you a powerful chest.

Number Of Repetitions

Beginner: 10 repetitions

Intermediate: 20 repetitions

Advanced: 40 repetitions

How To Perform The Exercise

1. Sit down on the edge of a chair.
2. Put your feet together while you spread your knees apart.
3. Place your hands on the outside of your knees. This is the starting position.
4. Use your hands to press your knees together. Your knees will offer resistance.
5. If you are doing the movement correctly you should feel tension in your pectoral muscles.

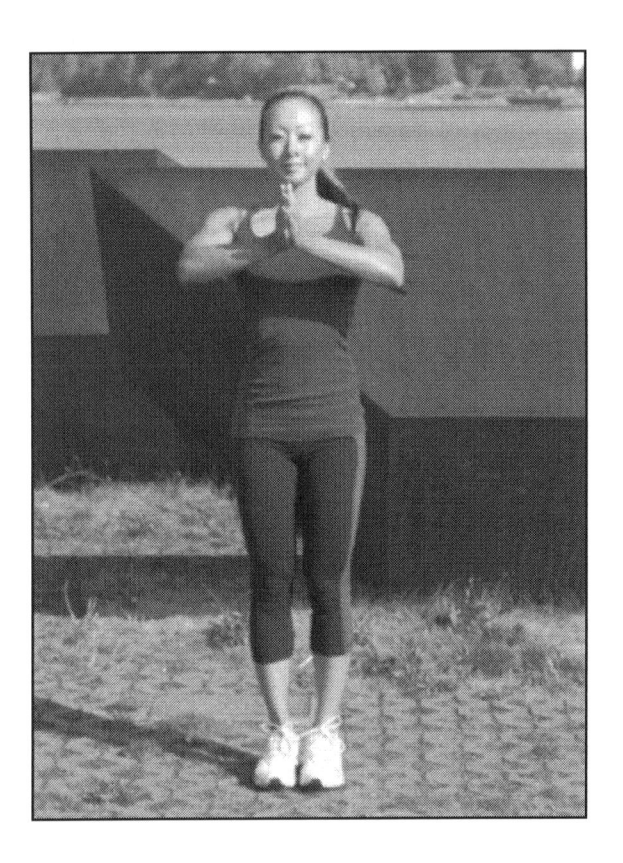

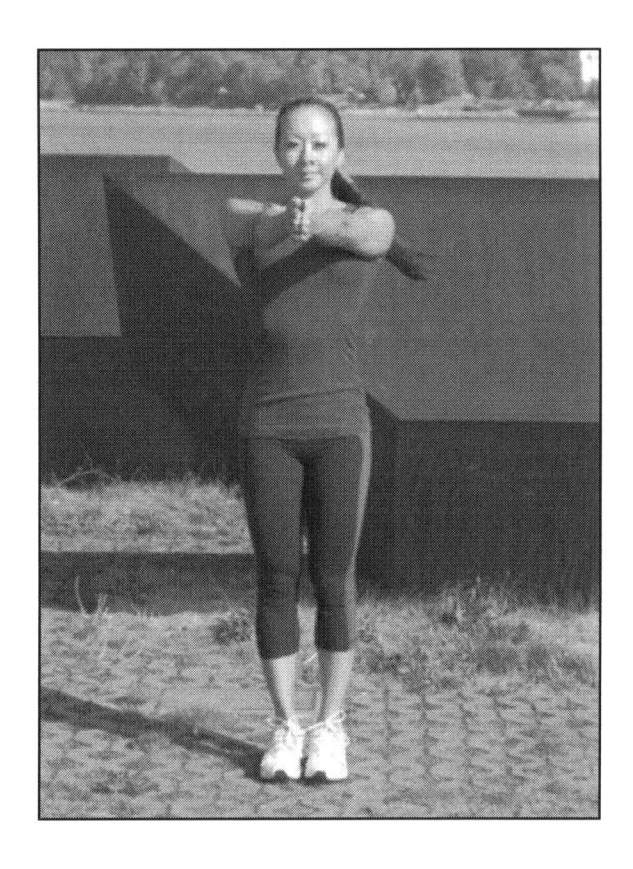

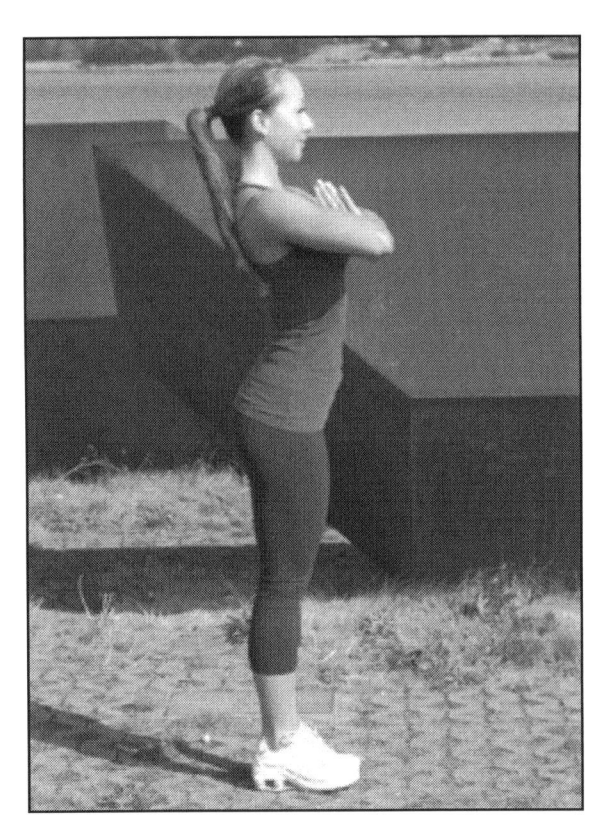

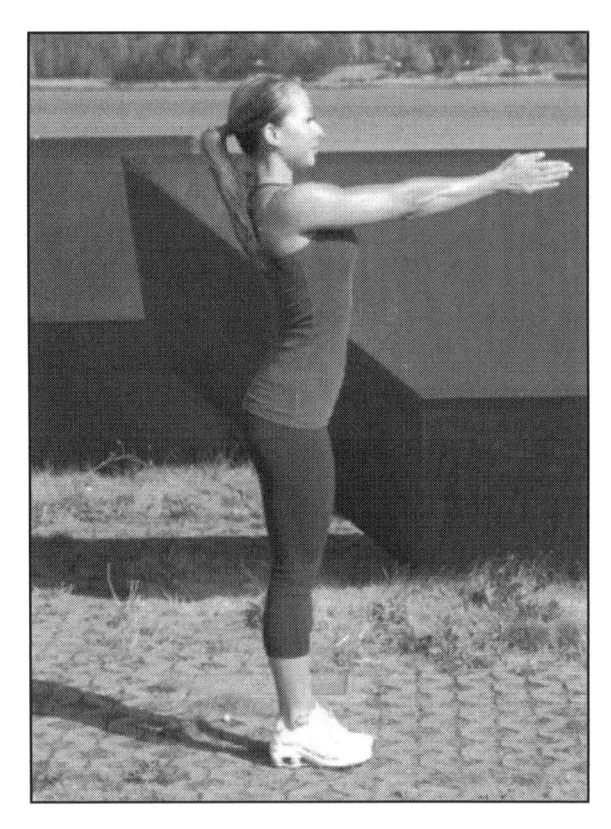

Copyright © 2010 David Nordmark. All rights reserved.
www.animal-kingdom-workouts.com

Page 26

Chest Presses

This exercise will help you further define your chest muscles.

Number Of Repetitions

Beginner: 10 repetitions

Intermediate: 20 repetitions

Advanced: 40 repetitions

How To Perform The Exercise

1. Put your hands together at mid chest level with your fingers pointed upwards. This is the starting position.
2. Perform the following simultaneously. Press your palms together while your rotate your fingers away from you. At the same time extend your arms straight out in front of you.
3. Bring your hands back to the starting position. Make sure you maintain the inward pushing tension against your palms. This counts as a single repetition.
4. Repeat for the required number of repetitions.

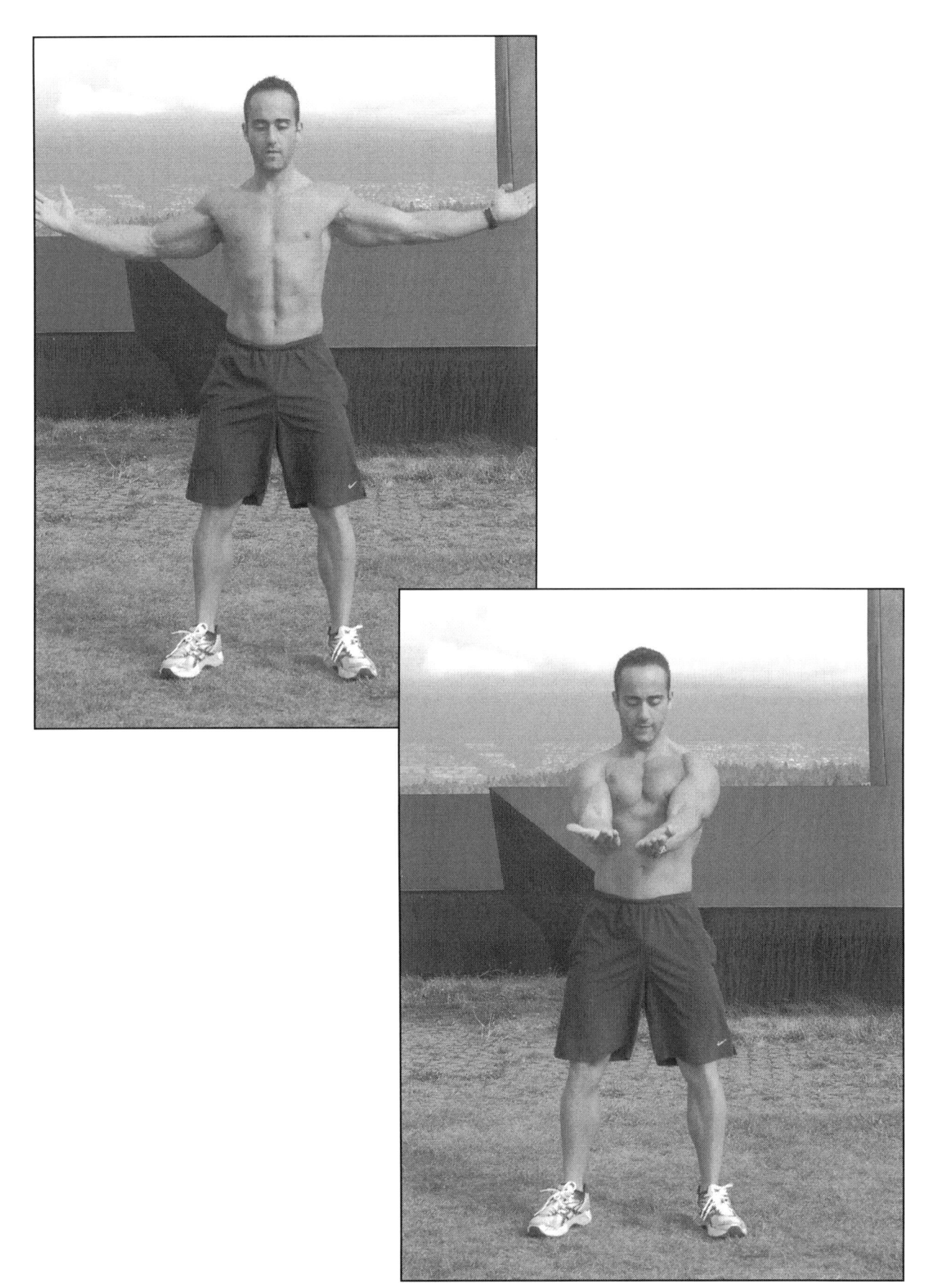

Chest Squeeze

This exercise needs to be done slowly and deliberately. Follow the breathing pattern and really focus on squeezing your chest muscles. This exercise will help add definition to your chest.

Number Of Repetitions

Beginner: 2 repetitions

Intermediate: 5 repetitions

Advanced: 10 repetitions

How To Perform The Exercise

1. Begin with your arms straight out to the sides and your feet shoulder width apart.
2. Breathe in through your nose for 3 to 4 seconds as you bring your arms together in front of you.
3. Hold your arms in front of you and squeeze your chest muscles. As you do so breathe out through your mouth for 7 to 12 seconds.
4. When you breathe out make sure your teeth are clenched and your tongue is on the roof of your mouth. You should be making a "SSSSSSS" sound, almost like a snake.
5. Breathe in through your nose again as you bring your arms apart.
6. Repeat for the required number of repetitions.

Abdominal Exercises

For aesthetics everyone wants a flat stomach and a six-pack abs look. However, there's more to the abdominal than just looks. Strong abdominal muscles will not only help you maintain youthfulness and vigor but will enhance the functionality of every gland and organ in your trunk. They also aid in digestion and elimination. Note that if you want the 6 pack abs look you will need to watch your body fat level. For men this usually means less than 10% body fat and for women less than 14%.

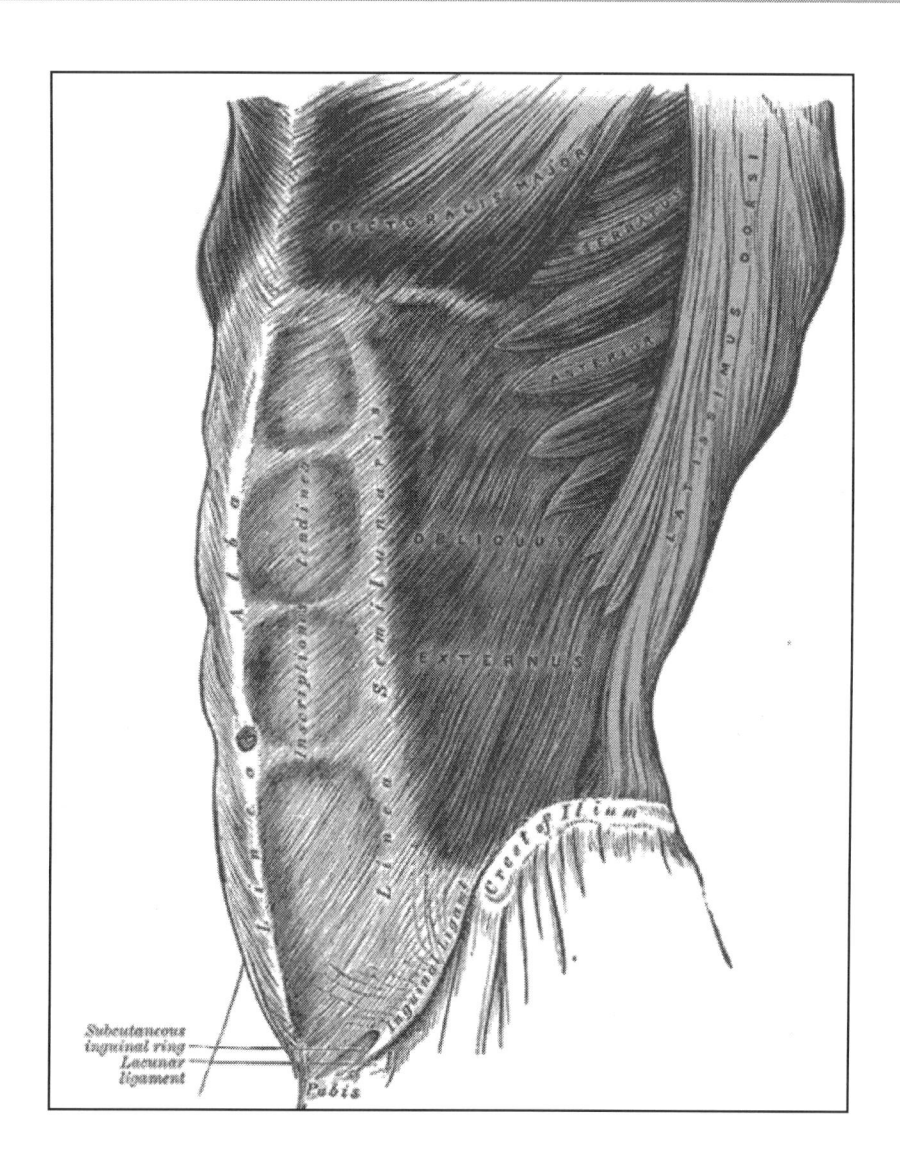

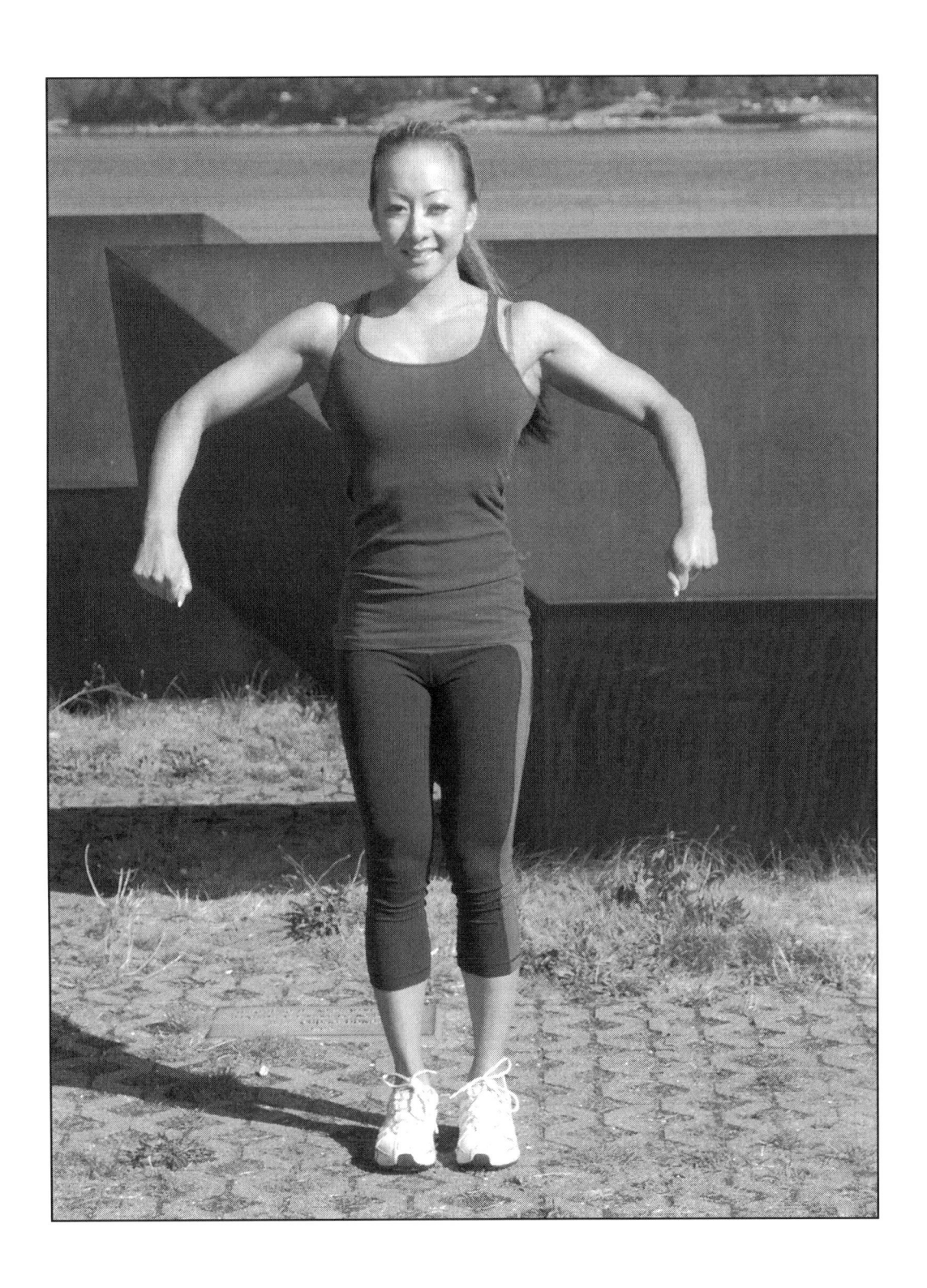

Isometric Stomach Flattener

This exercise, along with Iso-Vacuum, originally appeared in Power Isometrics. However, they are so effective I've decided to include them here as well. As an exercise, the Isometric Stomach Flattener is incredibly effective at working your stomach muscles and trimming your waistline. The reason it is so effective is that it works both your external and internal muscles. When you first try this exercise it's not uncommon to feel light-headed or dizzy. This feeling will pass with practice.

1. Stand up tall and straight with your hands by your sides.
2. Take a deep breath by breathing in through your nose for 3 to 4 seconds. Suck your stomach in as you do so.
3. Contract your abdominal muscles in as hard as you can for 7 to 12 seconds as you breathe out through your mouth making a "ssssssss" sound. For this contraction, imagine that your abdominal muscles are like a towel that you're wringing out.
4. While still keeping your stomach muscles sucked in, relax the tension as you breathe in gently for 3 to 4 seconds.
5. Repeat this process until you have completed 10 reps. Do NOT relax your stomach muscles until you have completed all 10 reps.

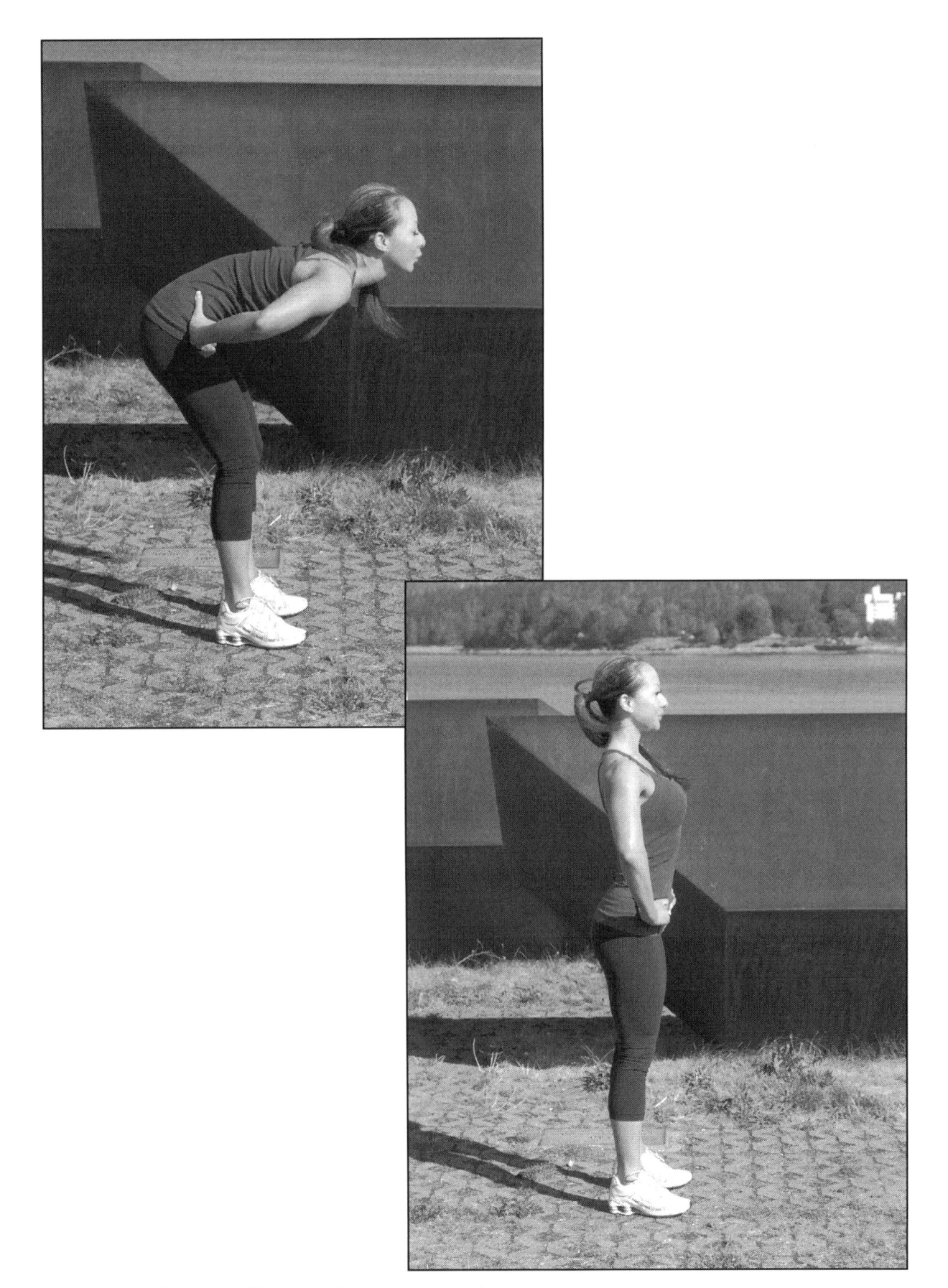

Copyright © 2010 David Nordmark. All rights reserved.
www.animal-kingdom-workouts.com

The Iso-Vacuum

Along with the Isometric Stomach Flattener, this exercise will reduce your waistline and improve the functioning of your digestive system. The deep breathing that accompanies this exercise will also energize you. Make sure you only perform this exercise on an empty stomach.

1. Stand straight up with your feet wider than shoulder-width apart.
2. Bend over at the waist (try to keep your back straight) while exhaling all of the air from your lungs.
3. Once you have bent over and breathed out the maximum amount of air that you can, suck your stomach in with as much force as possible.
4. Hold this contraction in your stomach and slowly stand up straight.
5. Hold this position, standing up straight with your stomach sucked in and no air in your lungs, for 7 seconds.
6. Inhale through your nose and slowly relax.
7. Repeat this exercise 10 times.

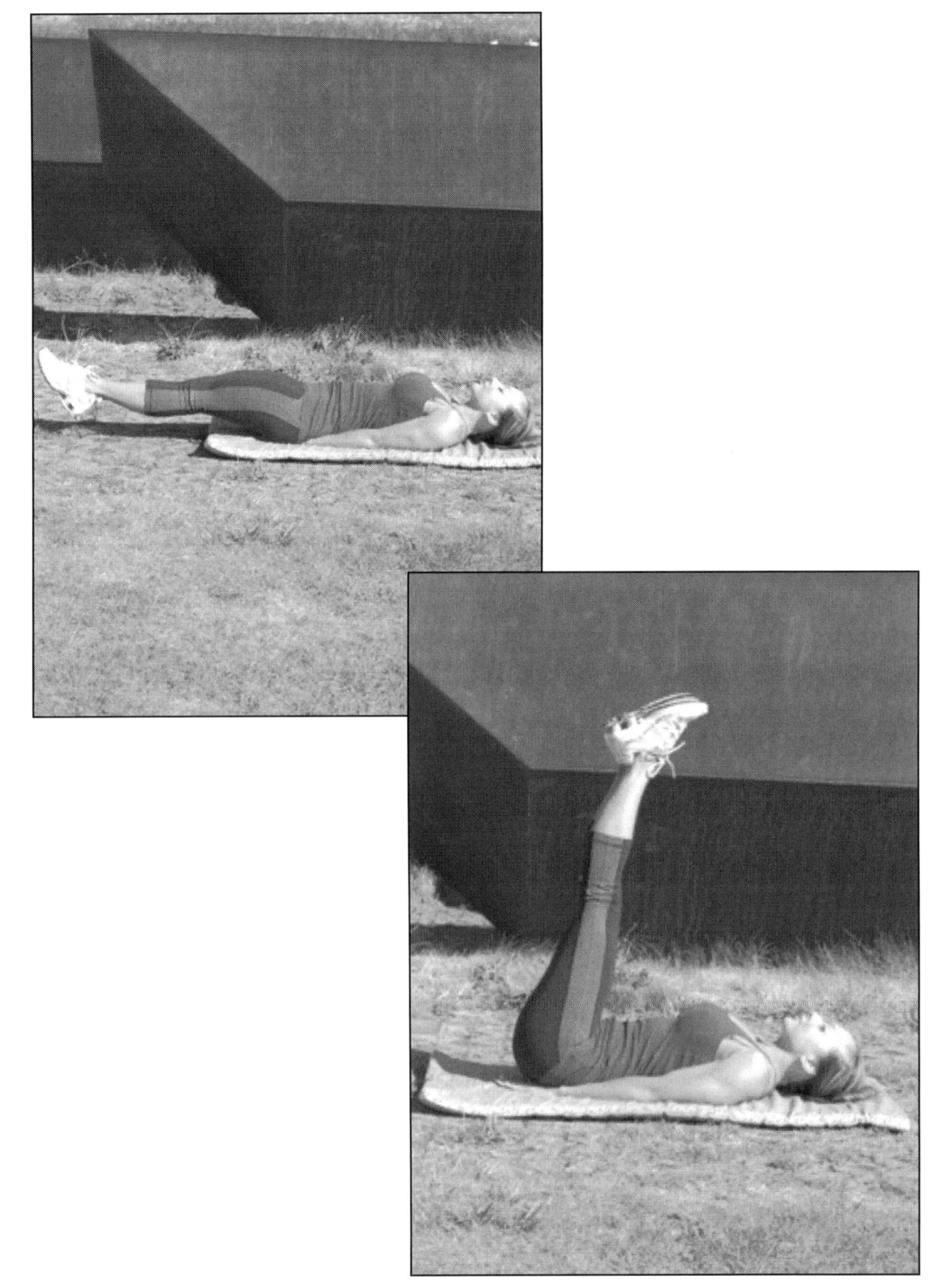

Leg Raise

This exercise will strengthen your abdominals, lower back and hip flexors. Like all abdominal exercises it will also massage your internal organs while increasing your circulation and aiding in the digestive process.

Number Of Repetitions

Beginner: 15 repetitions
Intermediate: 30 repetitions
Advanced: 60 repetitions

How To Perform The Exercise

1. Lie flat on the ground with your palms face down on the floor just below your lower back. Position your hands so that your lower back is supported and comfortable.
2. Inhale through your nose as you raise your legs up so that they are perpendicular to the floor.
3. Keep your legs straight at all times.
4. Make sure you move your legs with control. You want your abdominals doing the work, not gravity.
5. Lower your legs and repeat.

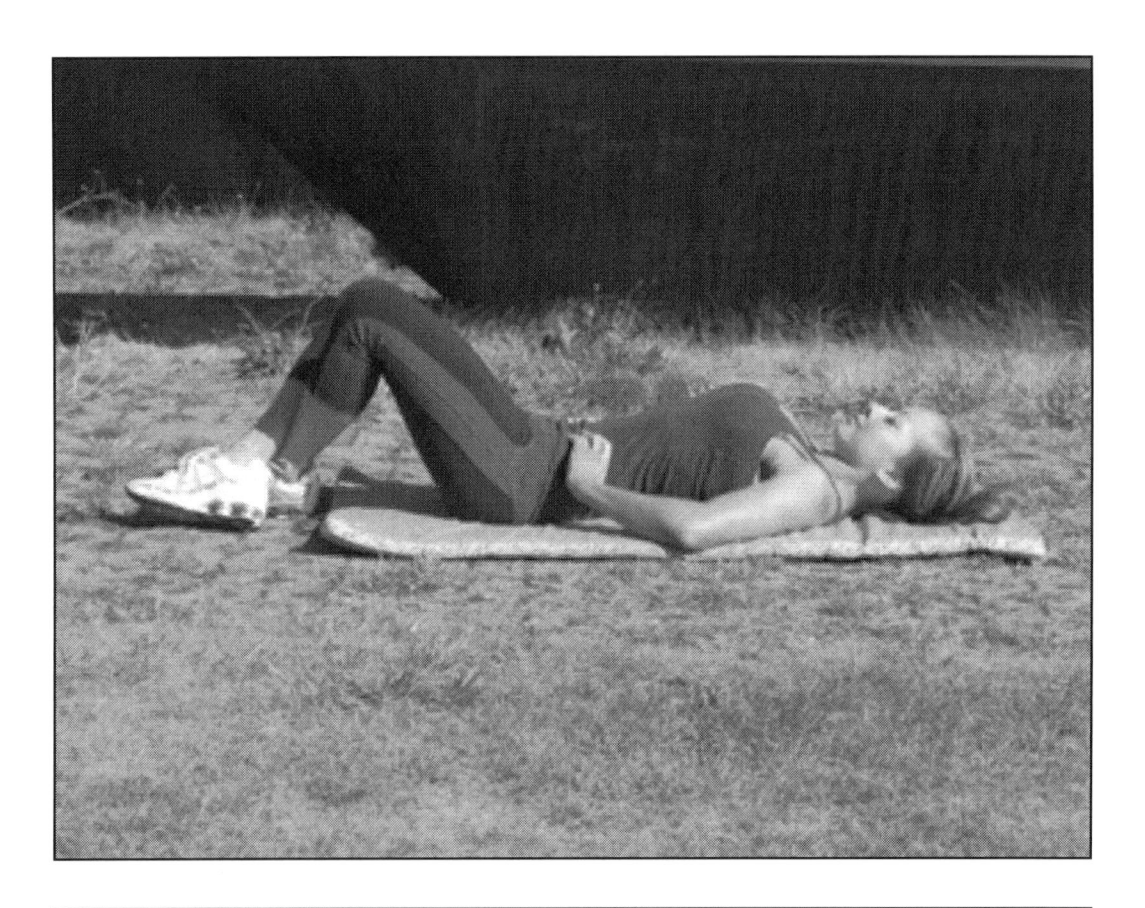

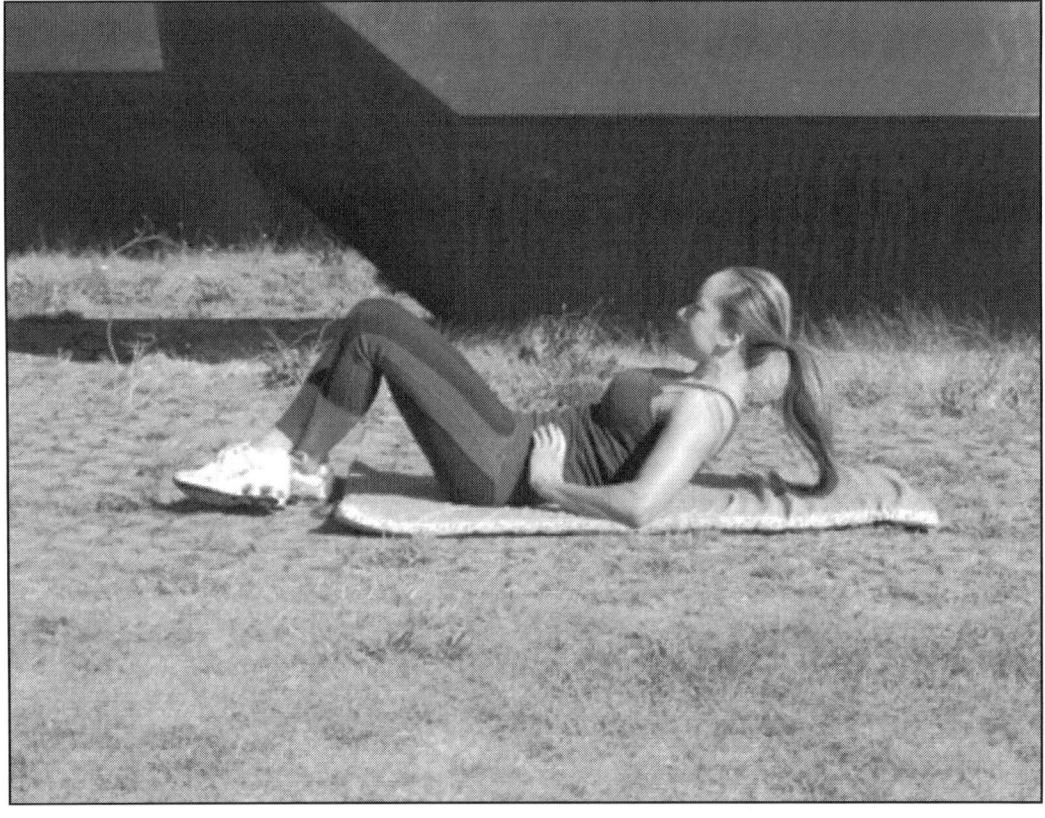

Concentrated Sit-Ups

Concentrated sit ups are a sit up variation that I prefer as they are easier on the lower back. Always remember to perform this movement slowly and deliberately. Never jerk your torso up or down. Your abdominals get just as much work during the backwards roll as when you are curling your spine upwards. It's all about using your abdominals to resist gravity as opposed to letting momentum do the work.

Number Of Repetitions

Beginner: 15 repetitions
Intermediate: 30 repetitions
Advanced: 60 repetitions

How To Perform The Exercise

1. Begin by lying flat on the floor with your knees bent, one ankle crossed over the other.
2. Bend your elbows and place your hands on your waist.
3. Begin slowly curling upwards starting with your neck and working down the spine.
4. Continue curling up until your lower back is barely touching the floor.
5. Pause at the top and then begin to curl your back down slowly.
6. Repeat for the required number of repetitions.

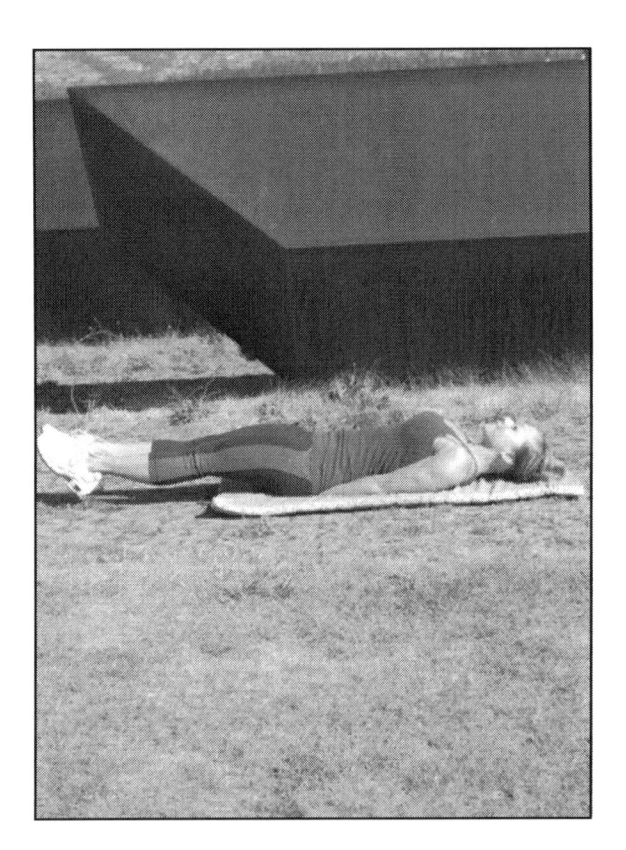

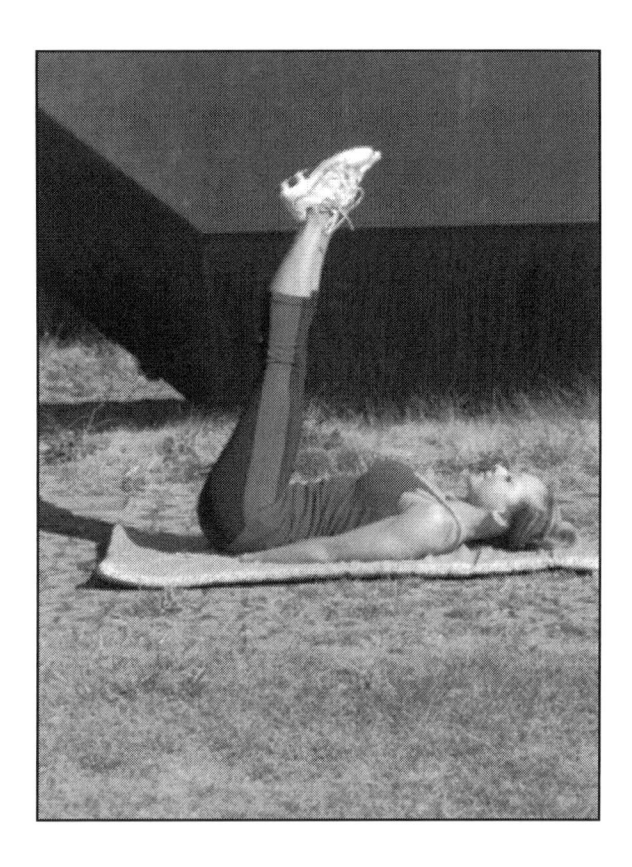

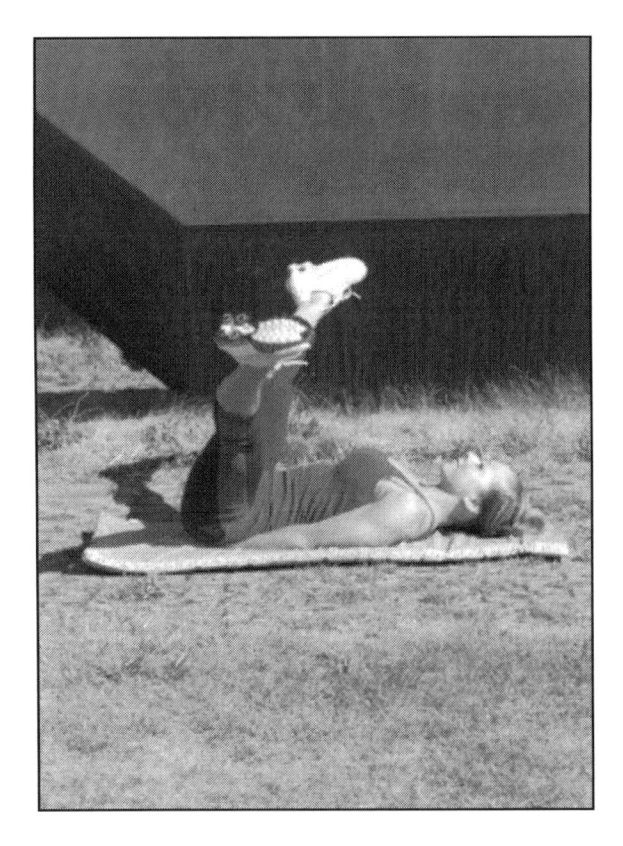

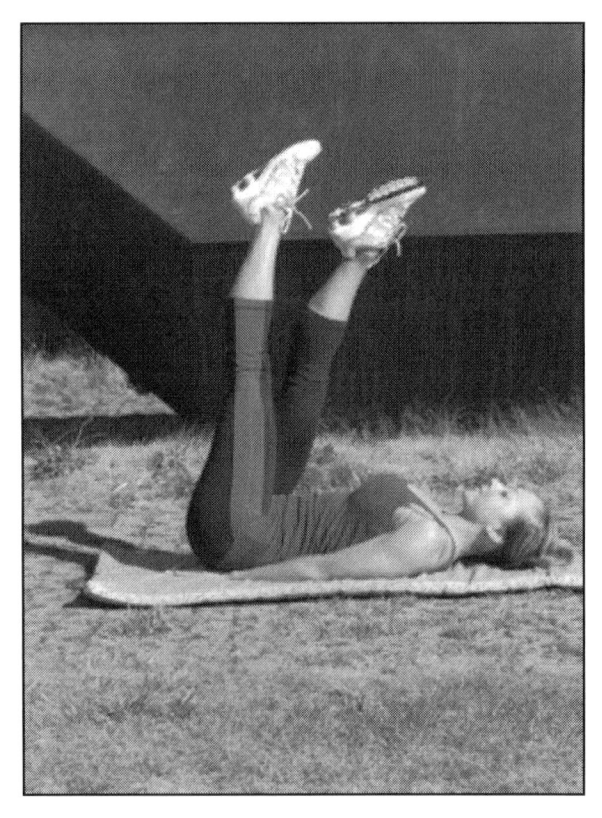

Copyright © 2010 David Nordmark. All rights reserved.
www.animal-kingdom-workouts.com

Leg Cross Raises

This exercise is a more advanced version of the Leg Raise. It involves spreading your legs apart in addition to raising your legs. This works your inner and outer thighs in addition to your hip flexors and abdominals.

Number Of Repetitions

Beginner: 10 repetitions
Intermediate: 20 repetitions
Advanced: 40 repetitions

How To Perform The Exercise

1. Lie flat on the ground with your palms face down on the floor just below your lower back.
2. Inhale through your nose as you raise your legs up so that they are perpendicular to the floor.
3. From this position, spread your legs apart then bring them back together crossing at the ankles.
4. Position your feet so that they are again side by side and then lower them to the ground.
5. Keep your legs straight at all times.
6. Alternate the ankle crosses (left behind right, right behind left) you perform with every movement.

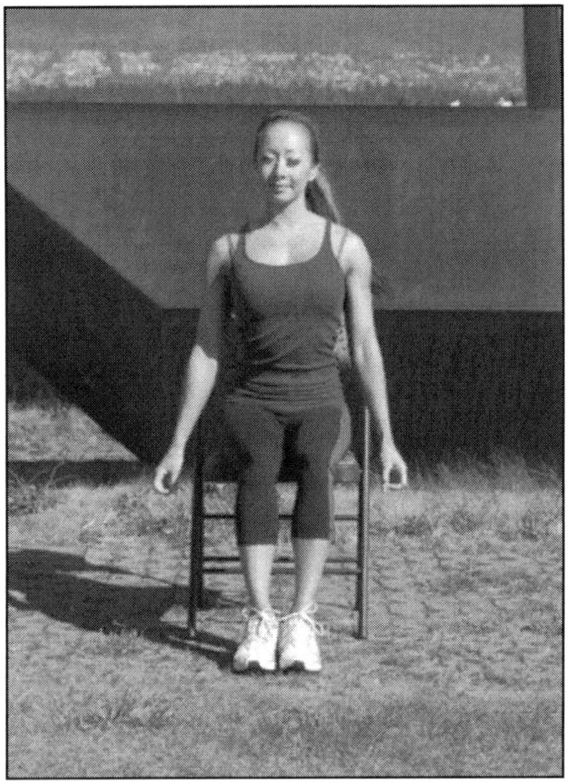

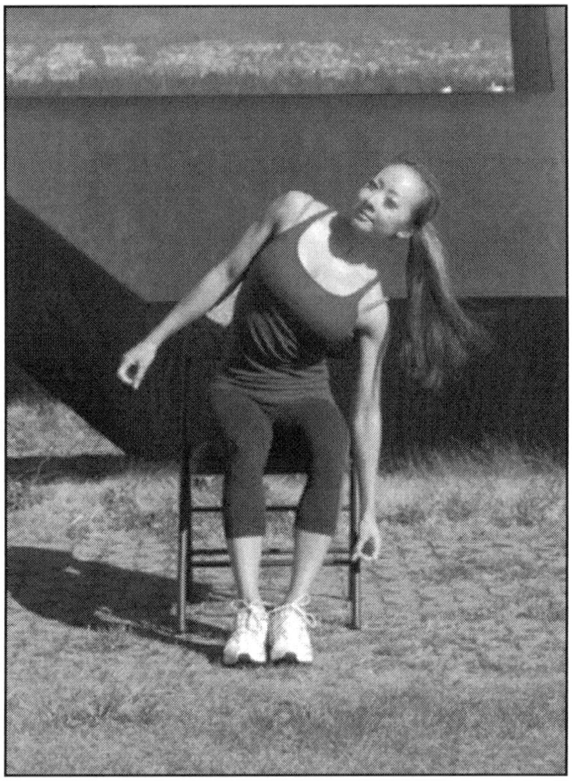

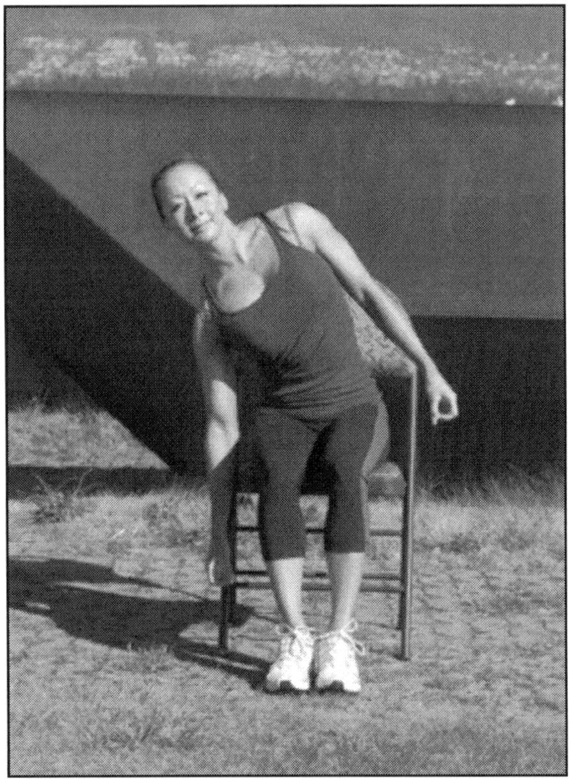

Side Bends

To really get the full benefit of this exercise you need to use your imagination. In your minds eye see yourself holding onto a heavy weight with one of your hands. As you bend over, imagine you are lowering the imaginary weight to the side. This will create a great deal of tension in your sides which will increase your strength and flexibility simultaneously.

Number Of Repetitions

Beginner: 10 (5 per side) repetitions
Intermediate: 20 (10 per side) repetitions
Advanced: 30 (15 per side) repetitions

How To Perform The Exercise

1. Sit down in an armless chair with your feet shoulder width apart and your arms straight down by your sides.
2. Slowly bring your right arm down to the side for a count of 2.
3. You should feel the right side of your waist contracting while the left side stretches.
4. Return to the original position for a count of 1.
5. Perform the required number of repetitions then switch sides.
6. Inhale through your nose as you bend to one side, exhale when you straighten your torso.

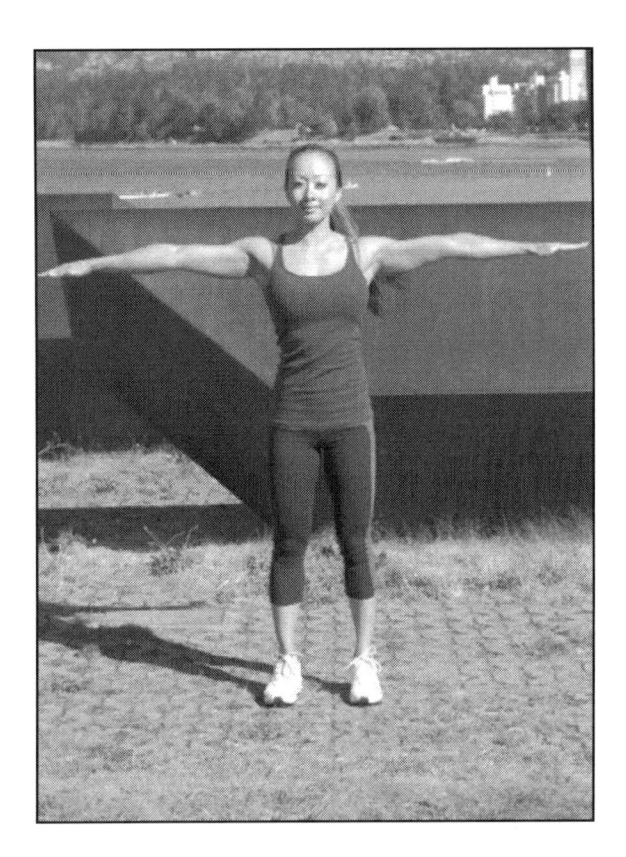

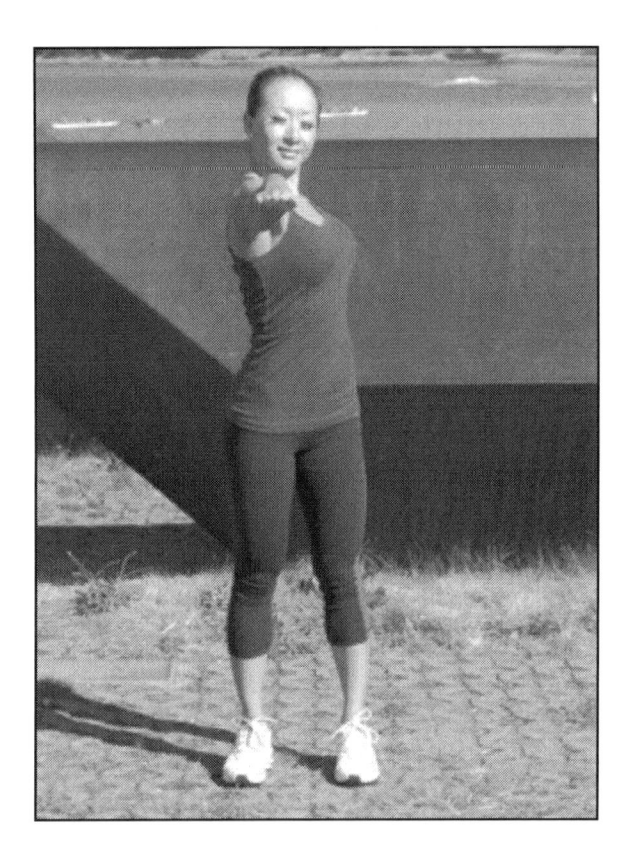

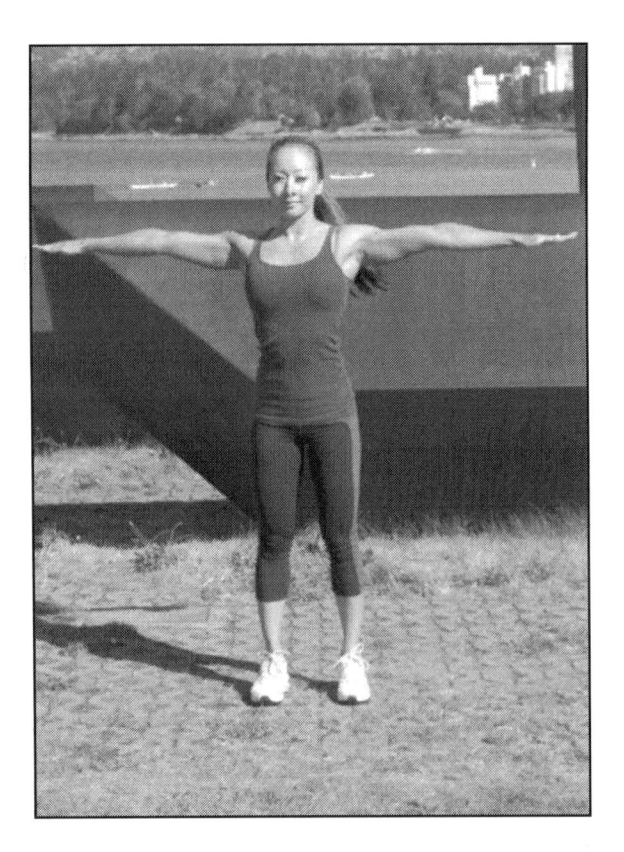

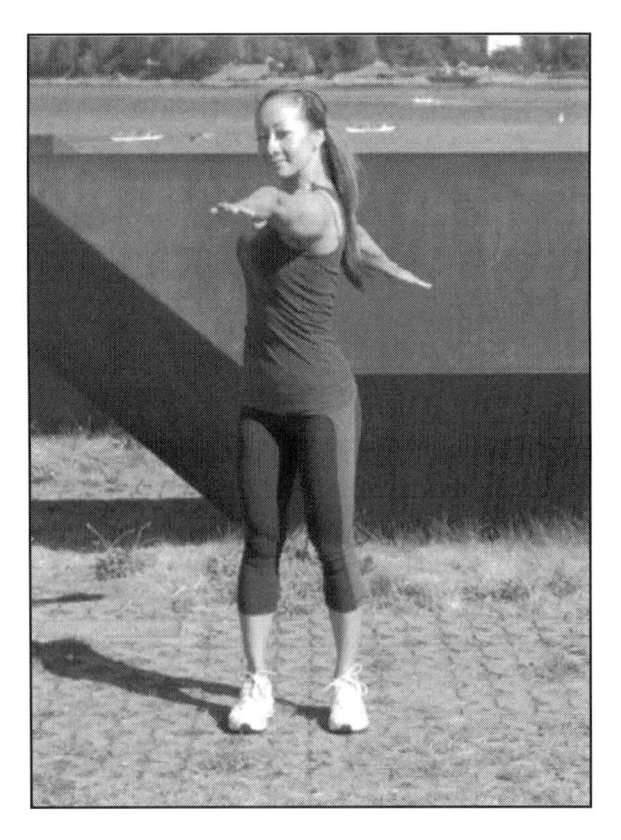

Copyright © 2010 David Nordmark. All rights reserved.
www.animal-kingdom-workouts.com

Page 44

Torso Twisting

Torso Twisting will strengthen your waist, abdomen, pelvis, lower back and pectorals. As you perform this motion make sure you keep your torso tight. You are not simply twisting from side to side. You are twisting with purpose and tension.

Number Of Repetitions

Beginner: 3 repetitions
Intermediate: 6 repetitions
Advanced: 9 repetitions

How To Perform The Exercise

1. Begin with your feet approximately 4 feet apart with your knees slightly bent.
2. Extend your arms out straight at shoulder level and your palms down.
3. Without moving your pelvis, twist your body slowly all the way to the left.
4. While twisting your body, ensure that your head is always looking forward.
5. Return to the starting position and then twist your body to the other side. This constitutes one repetition.

Exercises For The Neck

The neck muscles are incredibly important to train although most people ignore them. They shouldn't. A strong neck reduces the risk of injury and pain in this area. It can help reduce migraines and headaches as well as improve your posture. It can also improve the flow of blood to the brain, which will help keep you young. The neck development program that follows can help you with all of this..

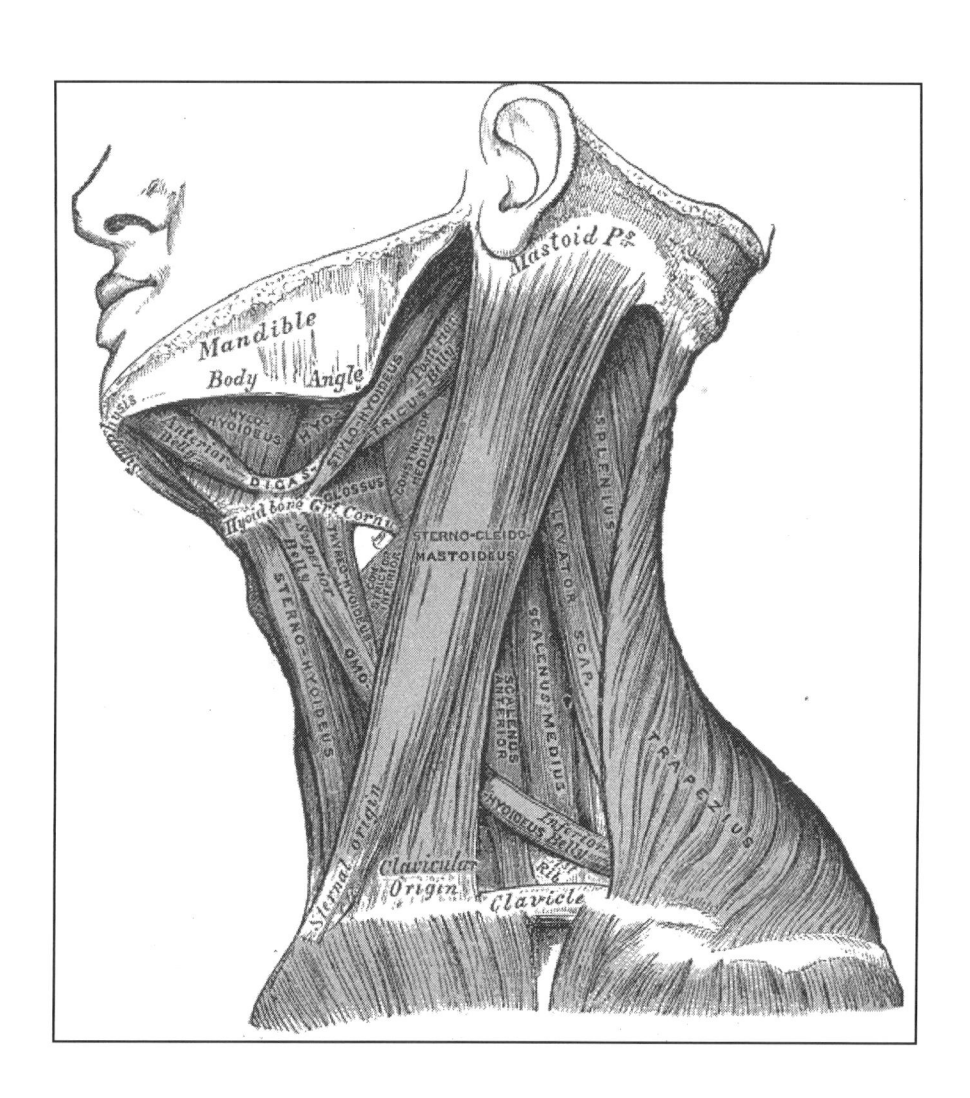

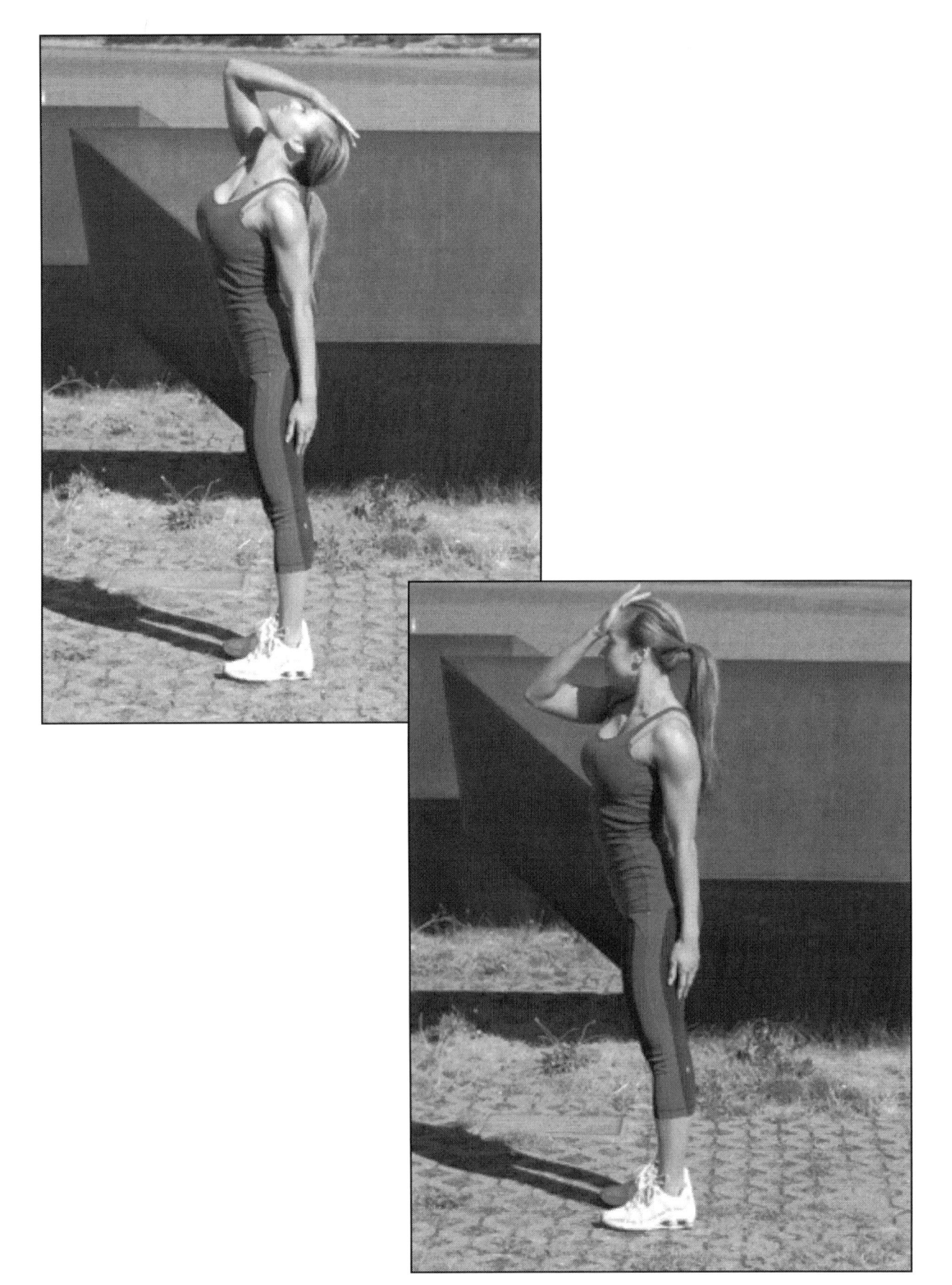

Copyright © 2010 David Nordmark. All rights reserved.
www.animal-kingdom-workouts.com

Page 48

Front Neck Conditioner

This exercise will tighten up the muscles in the front of your neck.

Number Of Repetitions

Beginner: 5 repetitions

Intermediate: 10 repetitions

Advanced: 20 repetitions

How To Perform The Exercise

1. Begin by standing straight up with your feet shoulder width apart.
2. Place the palm of one of your hands on your forehead.
3. Lean your head backwards so that you are looking at the ceiling.
4. Bring your head forward while using your hand to offer resistance.
5. Move your head slowly and evenly for a count of 2.

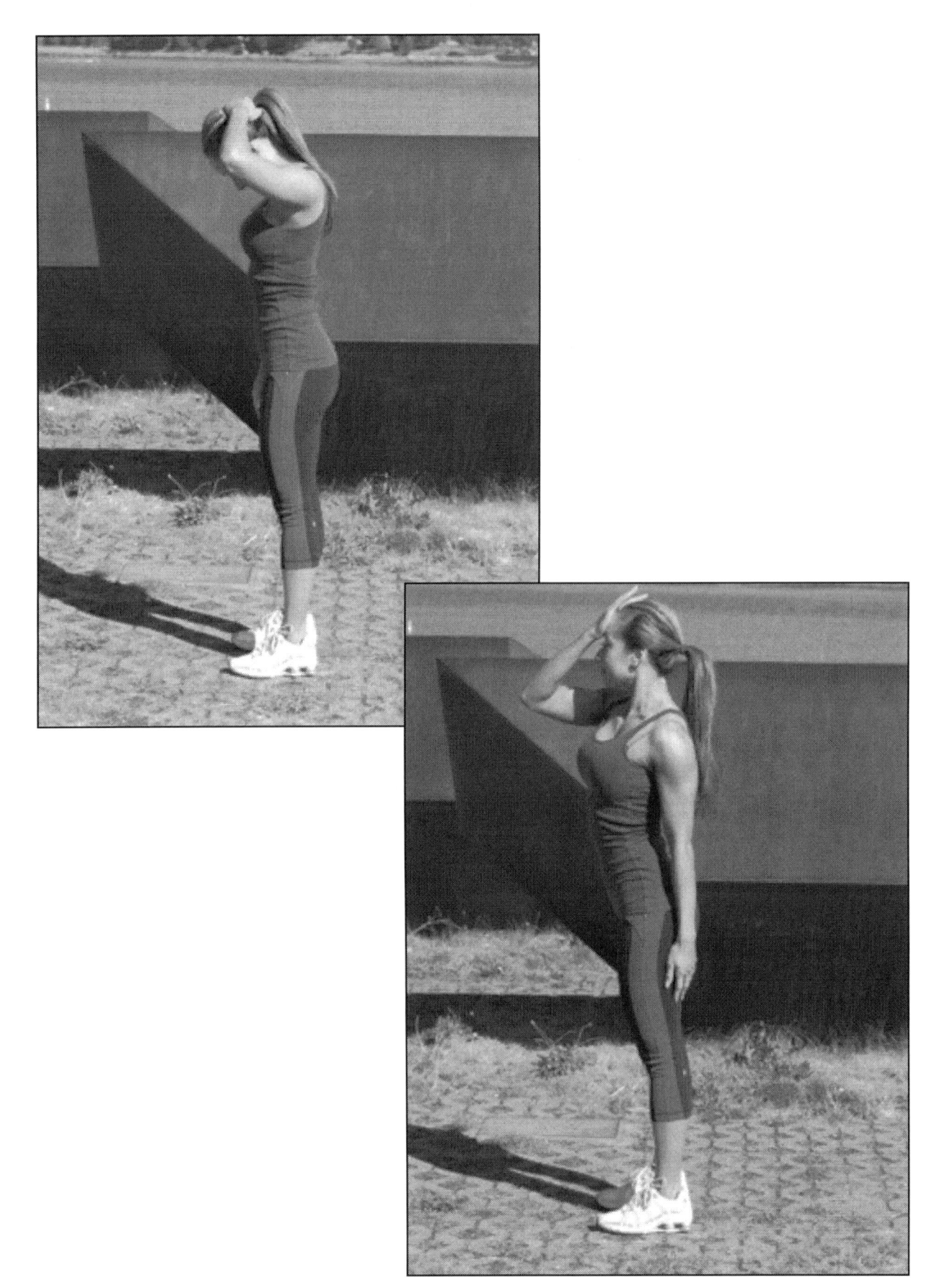

Copyright © 2010 David Nordmark. All rights reserved.
www.animal-kingdom-workouts.com

Page 50

Rear Neck Conditioner

This exercise will tighten and strengthen the muscles in the back of your neck.

Number Of Repetitions

Beginner: 5 repetitions

Intermediate: 10 repetitions

Advanced: 20 repetitions

How To Perform The Exercise

1. Begin by standing straight up with your feet shoulder width apart.
2. Place the palm of one of your hands on the back of your head.
3. Bring your chin forward so that it touches your chest.
4. Raise your head so that your neck is straight while using your hand for resistance.
6. Move your head slowly and evenly for a count of 2.

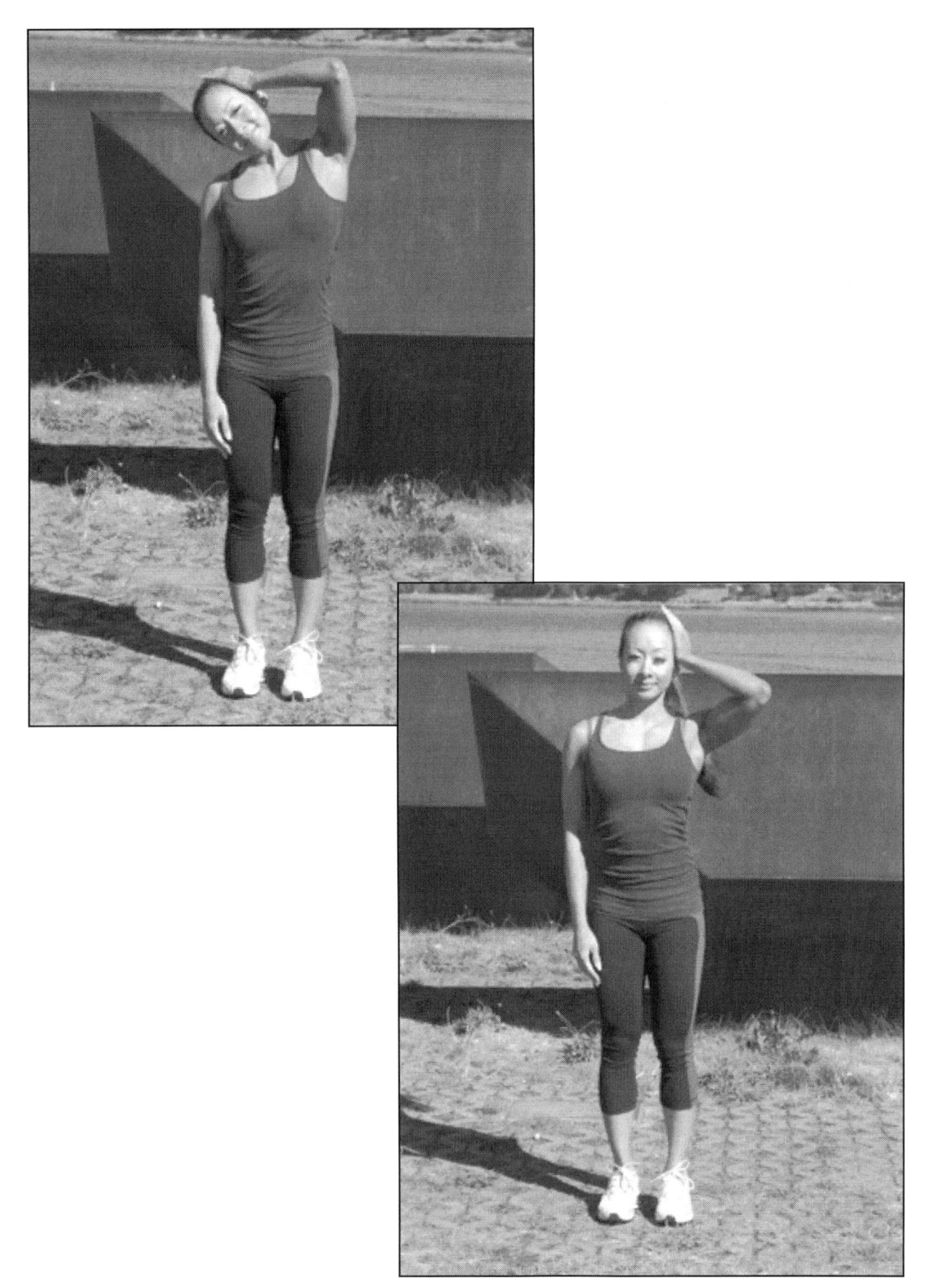

Side Neck Conditioner

This exercise will strengthen and tighten the muscles along the side of your neck.

Number Of Repetitions

Beginner: 10 (5 per side) repetitions

Intermediate: 20 (10 per side) repetitions

Advanced: 40 (20 per side) repetitions

How To Perform The Exercise

1. Begin by standing straight up with your feet shoulder width apart.
2. Place the palm of your right hand onto the side of your head. This is the beginning neutral position.
3. Lower your head to the left shoulder.
4. Raise your head back to the neutral position while using your right hand for resistance.
5. Once you have completed this exercise for one side of your neck repeat with the opposite side.
6. Move your head slowly and evenly for a count of 2.

Copyright © 2010 David Nordmark. All rights reserved.
www.animal-kingdom-workouts.com

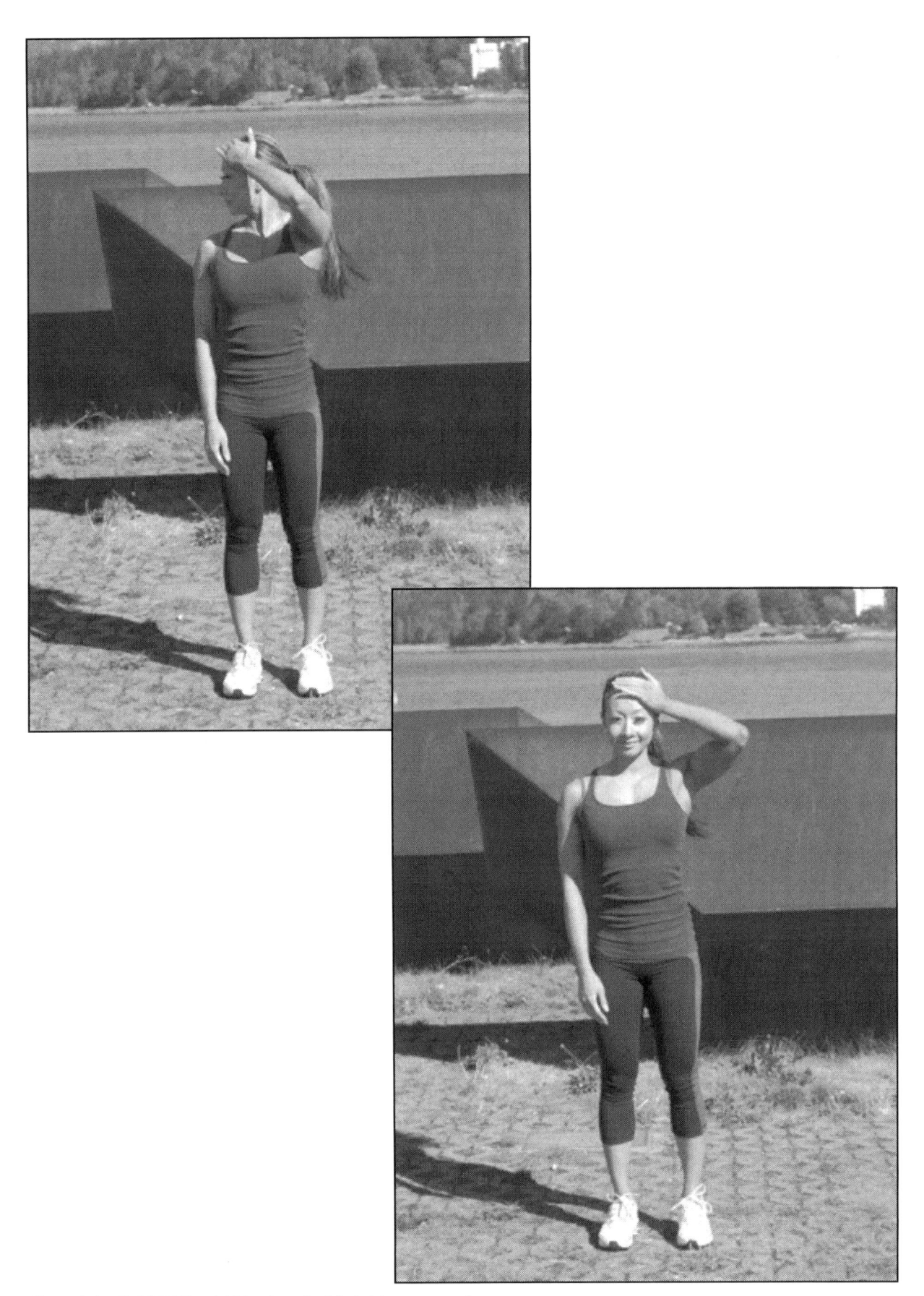

Copyright © 2010 David Nordmark. All rights reserved.
www.animal-kingdom-workouts.com   Page 54

Side Neck Twist

This exercise will strengthen and tighten the muscles along the side of your neck that are responsible for rotating your head.

Number Of Repetitions

Beginner: 10 (5 per side) repetitions

Intermediate: 20 (10 per side) repetitions

Advanced: 40 (20 per side) repetitions

How To Perform The Exercise

1. Begin by standing straight up with your feet shoulder width apart.
2. Place the palm of your right hand on your right temple. This is the beginning or neutral position.
3. Turn your head to the left.
4. Turn your head back to the neutral position, using your right hand to provide resistance.
5. Once you have completed this exercise for one side of your neck repeat with the opposite side.

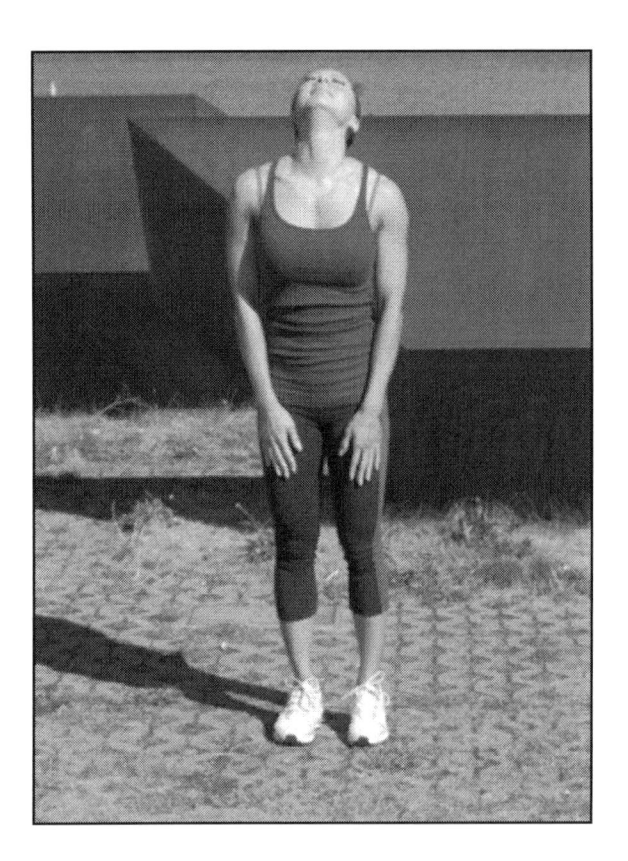

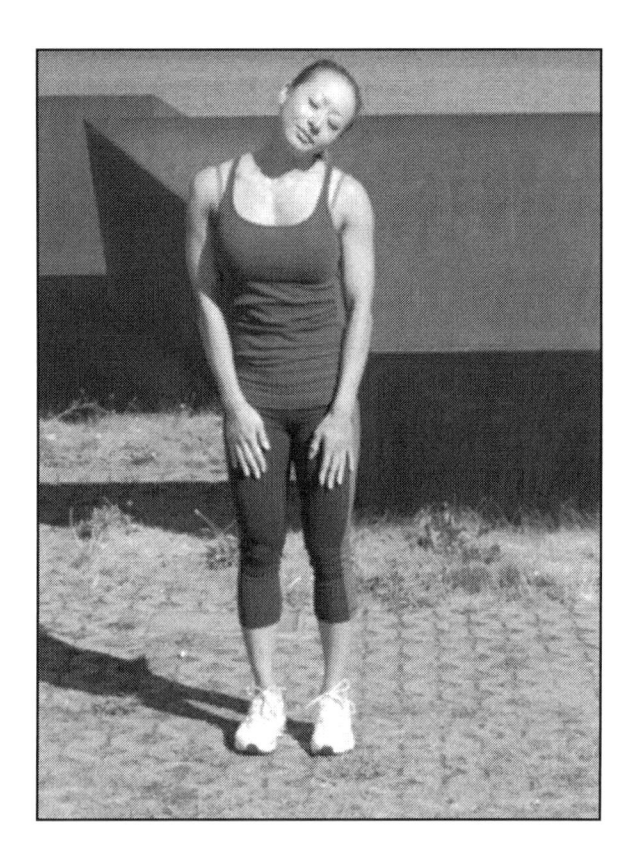

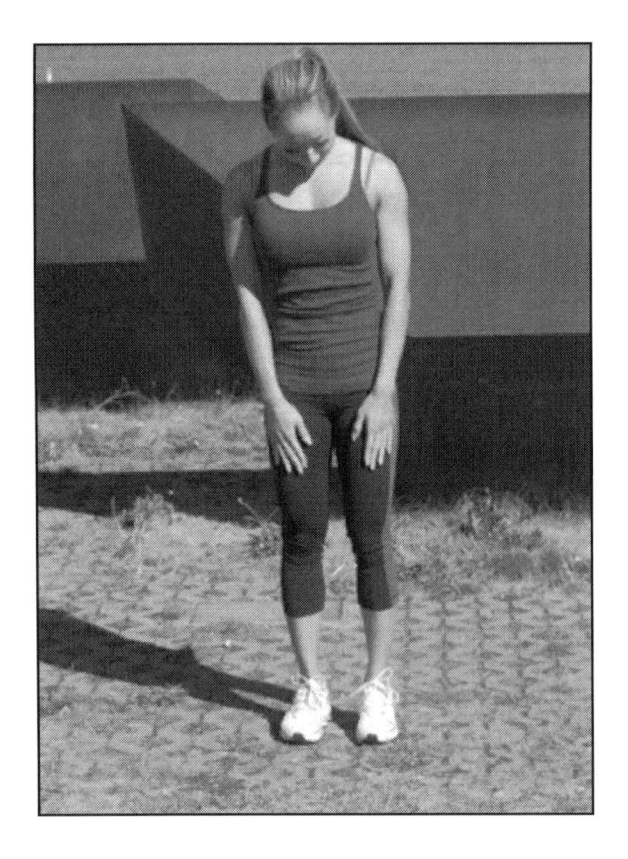

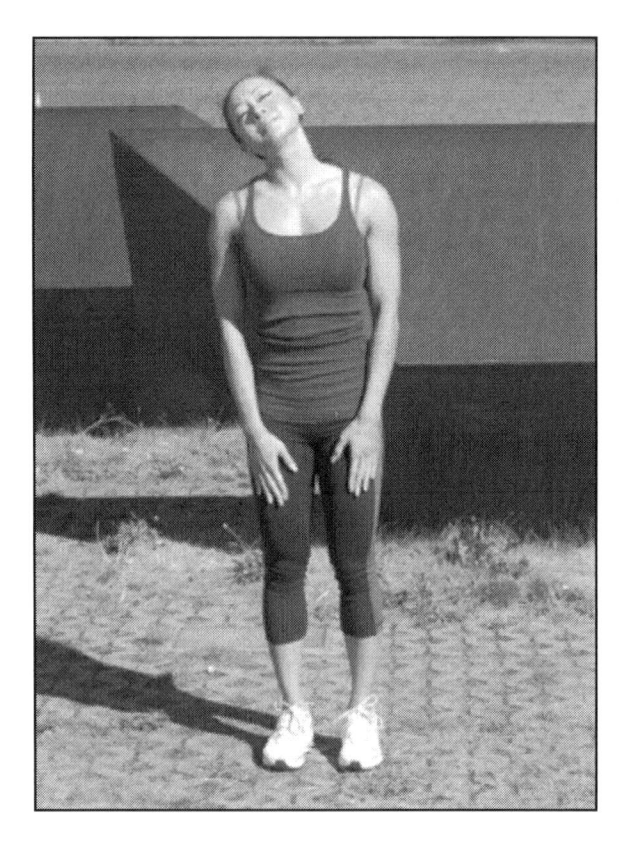

Neck Rotations

This exercise will stretch and loosen all of the muscles in the neck.

Number Of Repetitions

Beginner: 10 (5 each way) repetitions

Intermediate: 20 (10 each way) repetitions

Advanced: 40 (20 each way) repetitions

How To Perform The Exercise

1. Begin by standing straight up with your feet shoulder width apart.
2. Bend your head backwards so that you are looking at the ceiling.
3. Now simply roll your head in a circular motion from one shoulder to the chest to the opposite shoulder and then back again.
4. One complete circular motion constitutes one repetition.
5. Once you have completed the required number of neck rotations one way repeat the motion in the opposite direction.

Shoulder Exercises

Strong, broad shoulders are considered desirable by both men and women. They can not only enhance your appearance but can also help you in any sport you play. The following exercises will help you build and sculpt your shoulders.

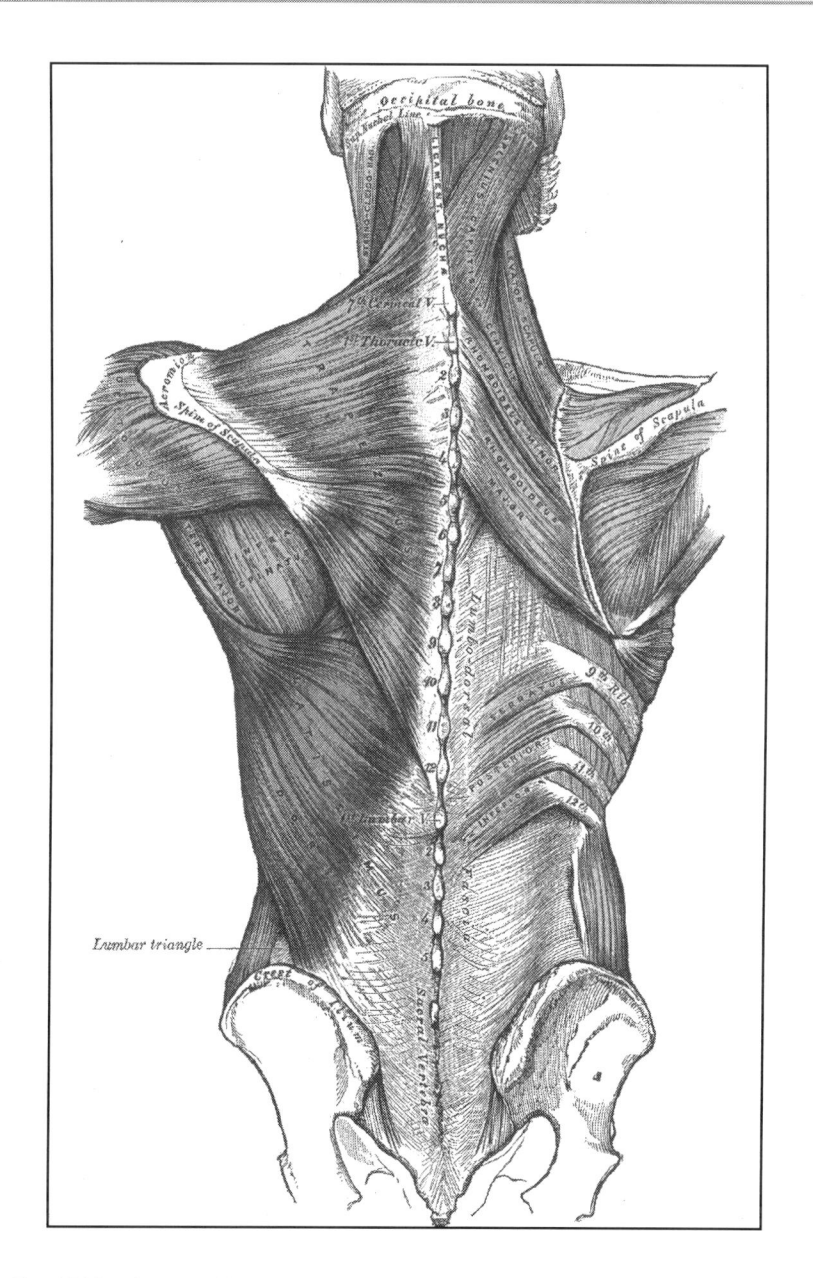

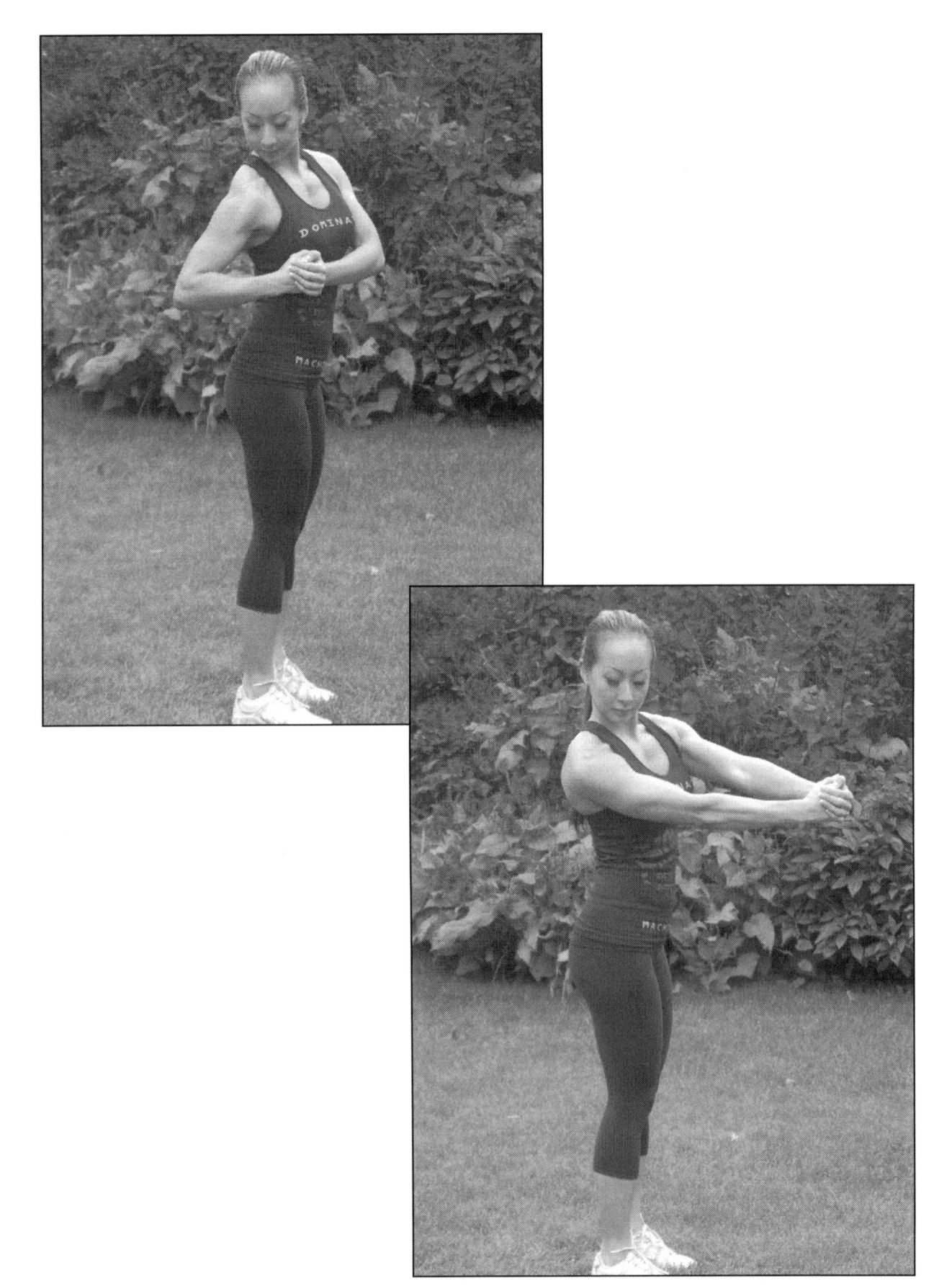

Copyright © 2010 David Nordmark. All rights reserved.
www.animal-kingdom-workouts.com

Page 60

Shoulder Pushes

Shoulder Pushes are an excellent exercise for strengthening and toning the shoulder muscles. This one really works those in the front of the shoulder, otherwise known as the Anterior Deltoid.

Number Of Repetitions

Beginner: 20 (10 per side) repetitions
Intermediate: 40 (20 per side) repetitions
Advanced: 80 (40 per side) repetitions

How To Perform The Exercise

1. Stand straight up with your feet shoulder width apart.
2. Make a fist with your right hand and place it by your right side.
3. Cover your right fist with the palm of your left hand.
4. Resisting with your left hand, press your right hand forward and then back.
5. Your should always feel a tension in your arms and shoulders. When you press forward the right arm is dominant, when you press backward the left is.
6. Once you have completed the required repetitions with your right hand repeat with your left.

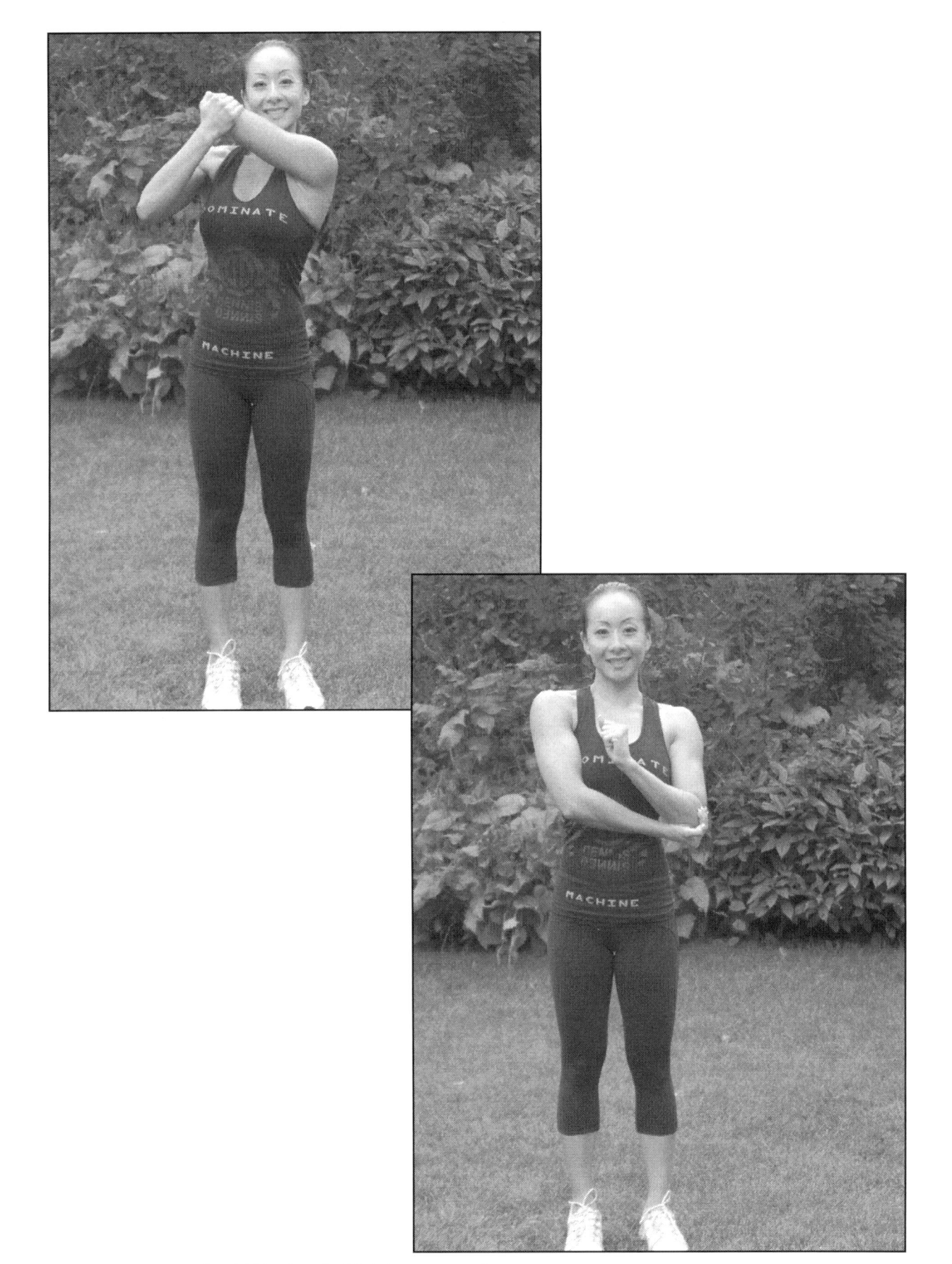

Copyright © 2010 David Nordmark. All rights reserved.
www.animal-kingdom-workouts.com

Page 62

Elbow Presses

Elbow Presses focus on the muscles in the rear of your shoulder, otherwise known as the Posterior Deltoid.

Number Of Repetitions

Beginner: 20 (10 per side) repetitions

Intermediate: 40 (20 per side) repetitions

Advanced: 60 (30 per side) repetitions

How To Perform The Exercise

1. Begin standing straight up with your feet shoulder width apart.
2. Raise up your right arm so that your right bicep is almost at your chin.
3. Bend your right arm so that your right hand is almost touching your left shoulder.
4. Place the palm of your left hand on your right elbow. This is the starting position.
5. Resisting with your left hand bring your right arm so that your right elbow is by your side.
6. Inhale as you press your right elbow down, exhale when you return to the starting position.

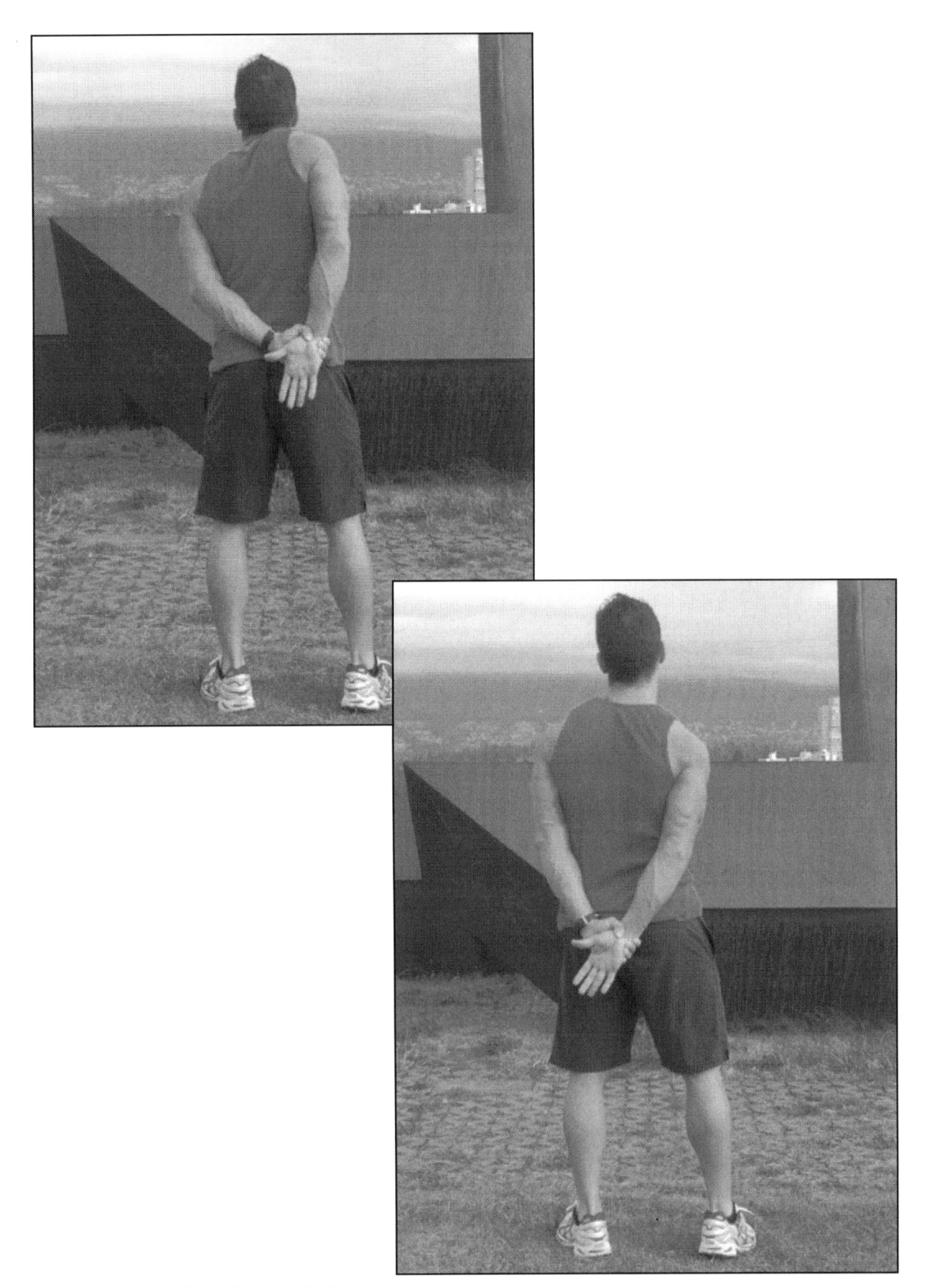

Copyright © 2010 David Nordmark. All rights reserved.
www.animal-kingdom-workouts.com

Shoulder Shrugs

This exercise will strengthen and promote flexibility along the top of your shoulders.

Number Of Repetitions

Beginner: 20 (10 per side) repetitions

Intermediate: 40 (20 per side) repetitions

Advanced: 60 (30 per side) repetitions

How To Perform The Exercise

1. Begin standing straight up with your feet shoulder width apart.
2. Bring your left arm behind you.
3. Grab the wrist of your left arm with your right hand. This is the starting position.
4. Shrug your left shoulder upwards while your right hand pulls downwards offering resistance.
5. For this one, you only want to offer resistance when you shrug your shoulder upwards. Relax when you return to the starting position.

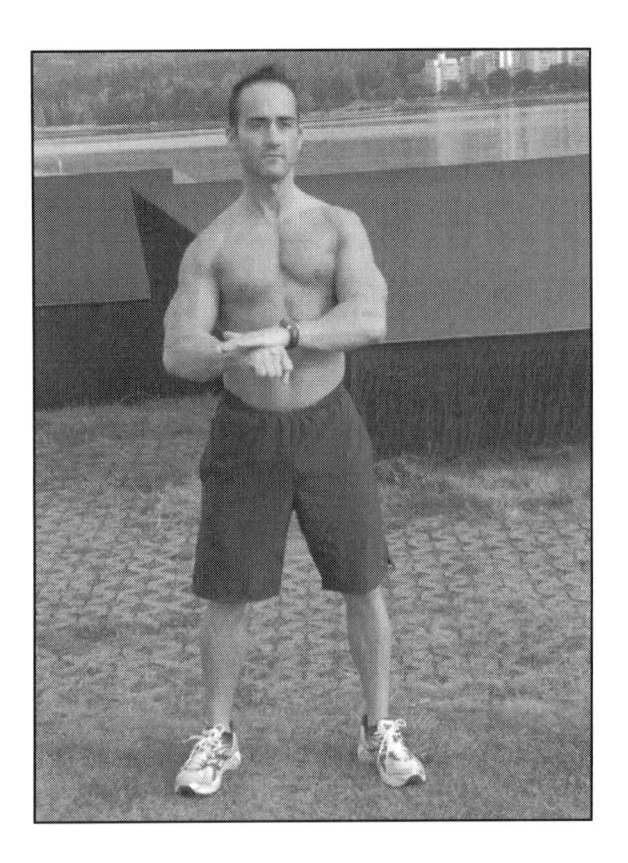

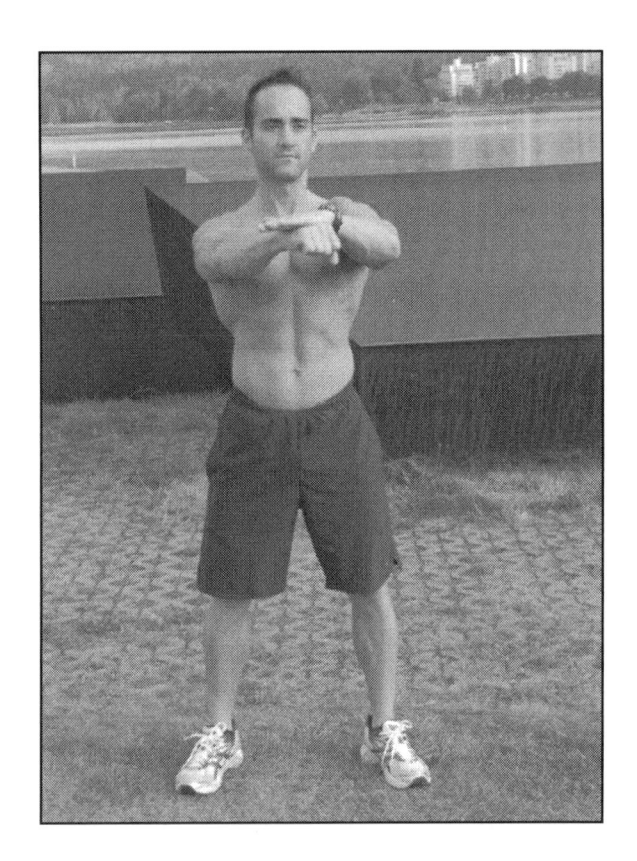

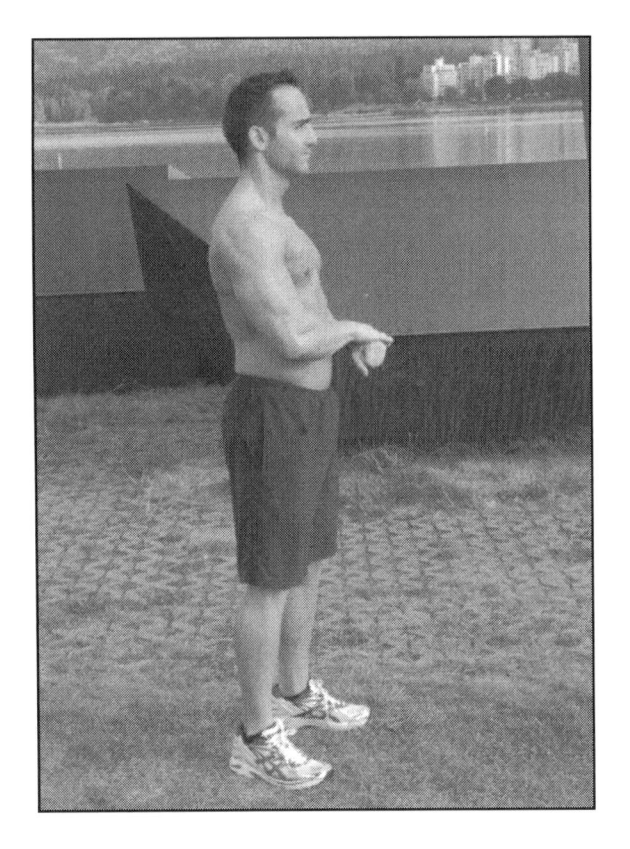

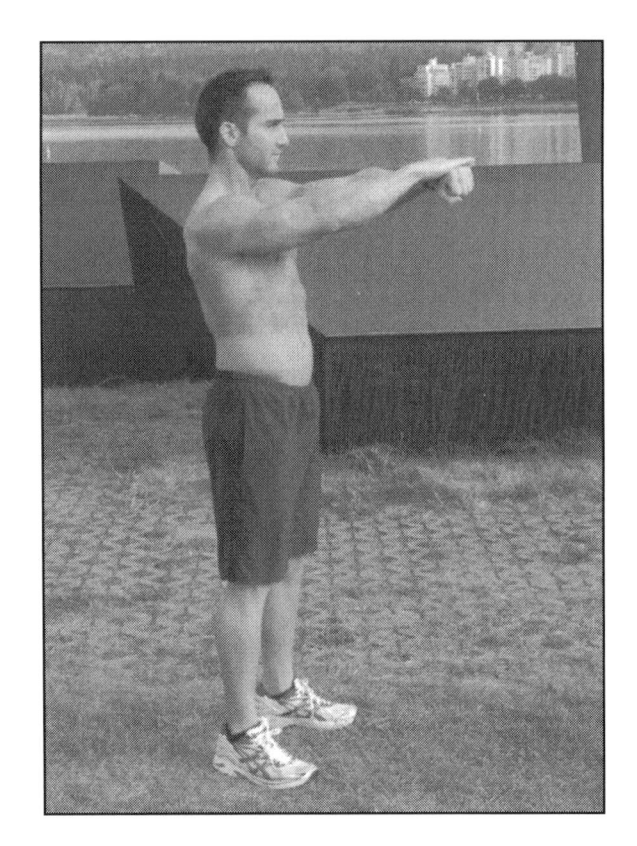

Shoulder Extensions

Shoulder Extensions work your entire shoulders, focusing on the front and top.

Number Of Repetitions

Beginner: 20 (10 per side) repetitions

Intermediate: 40 (20 per side) repetitions

Advanced: 80 (40 per side) repetitions

How To Perform The Exercise

1. Begin standing straight up with your feet shoulder width apart.
2. Make a fist with your right hand and place it on the left side of your waist. Your right arm should be flexed at a 90 degree angle.
3. Place your left hand over your right hand. This is the starting position.
4. Extend your right arm up and out. Upon completing the movement your right fist should be almost at your chin level.
5. Relax and return your arms to the starting position and repeat.
6. Once you have completed the required repetitions with your right hand repeat with your left.

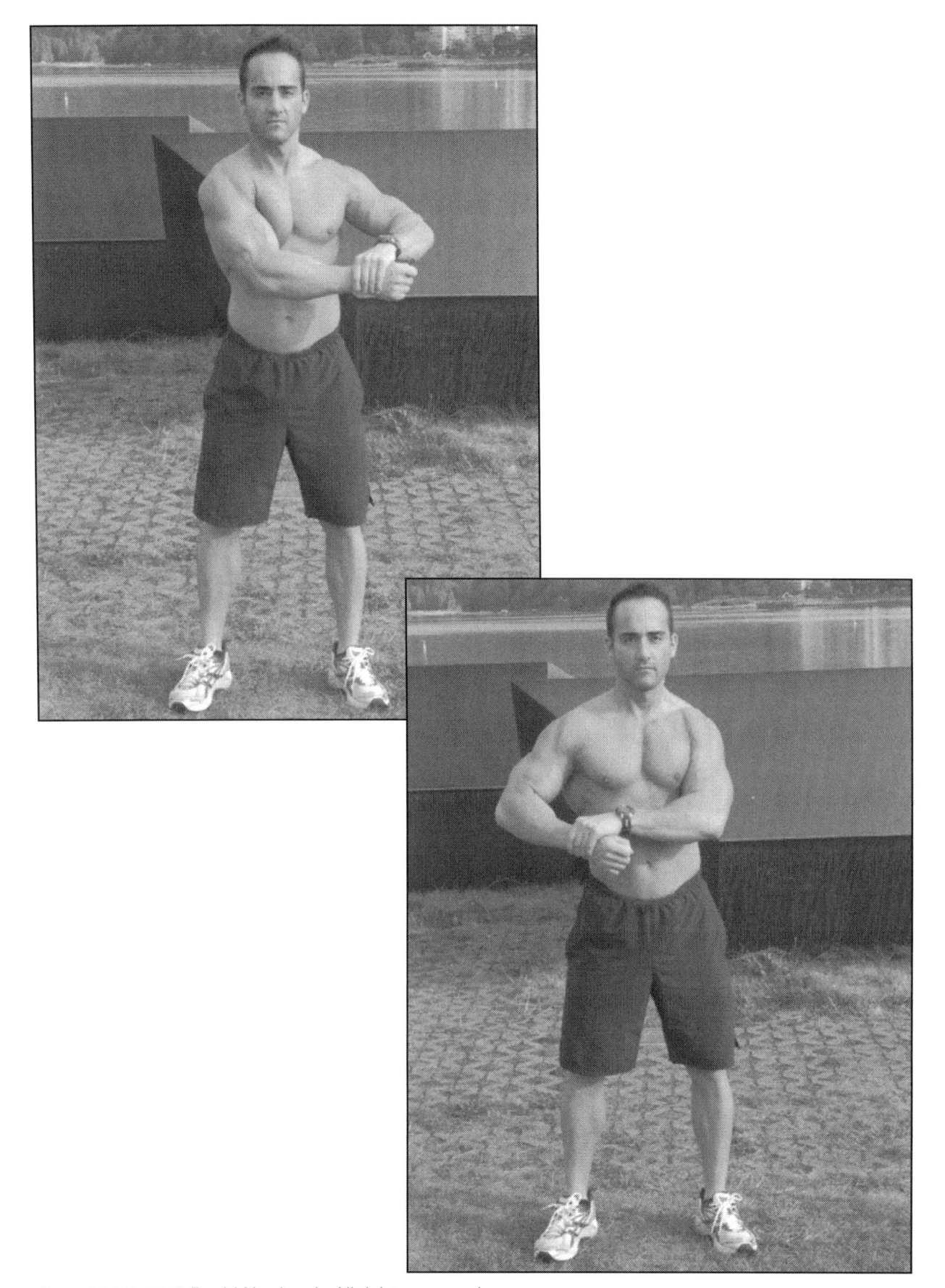

Shoulder Pulls

Shoulder Pulls are another fantastic overall shoulder developer.

Number Of Repetitions

Beginner: 20 (10 per side) repetitions

Intermediate: 40 (20 per side) repetitions

Advanced: 60 (30 per side) repetitions

How To Perform The Exercise

1. Begin standing straight up with your feet shoulder width apart.
2. Make a fist with your right hand with the palm up and place it on the left side of your waist.
3. Place your left hand over your right hand, grabbing it firmly. This is the starting position.
4. Resisting with your left hand pull your right arm out to the side.
5. Return your arms to the starting position and repeat offering resistance in both directions.
6. Once you have completed the required repetitions with your right arm repeat with your left.

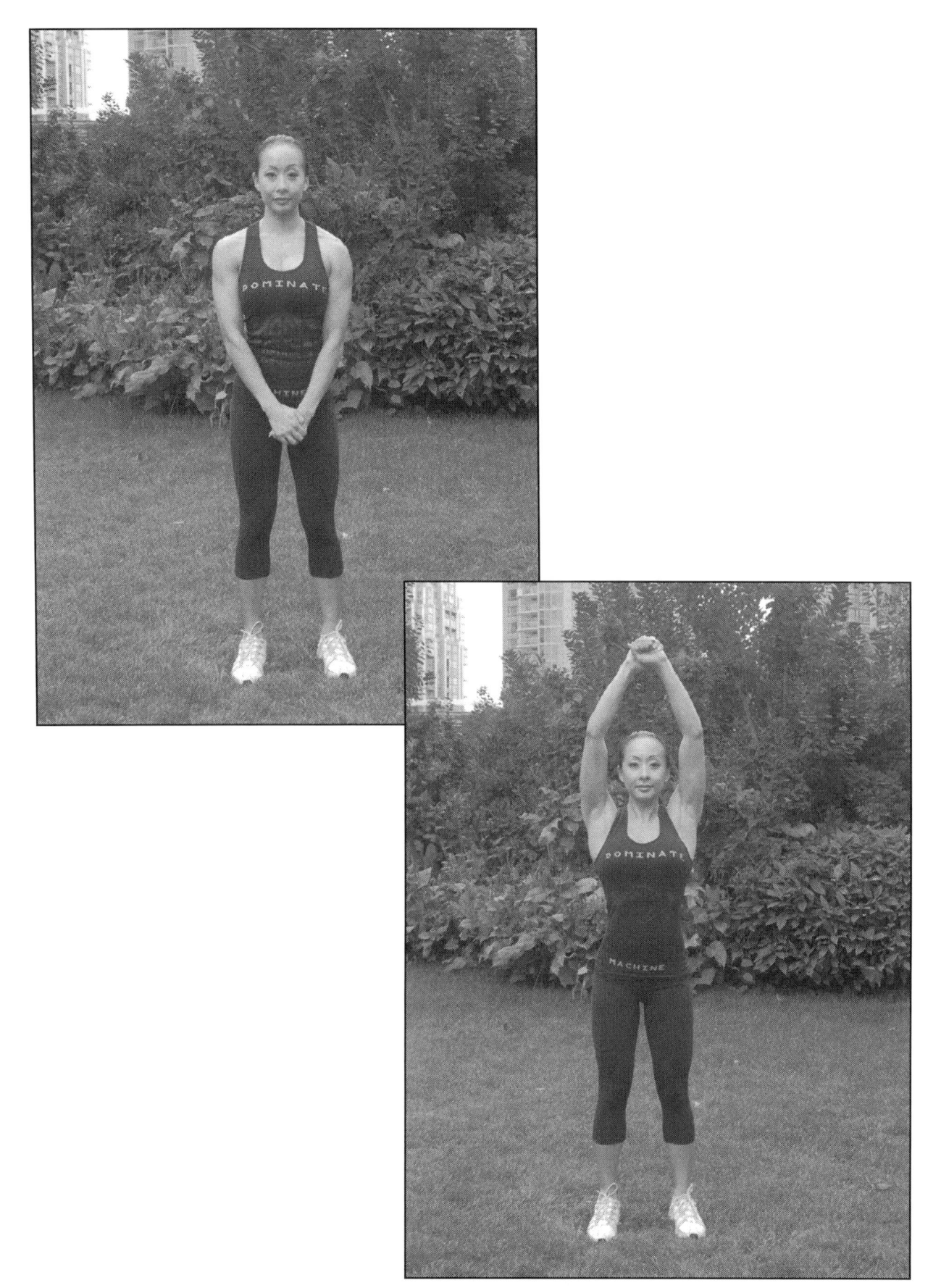

Shoulder Raises

Number Of Repetitions

Beginner: 20 (10 per side) repetitions

Intermediate: 40 (20 per side) repetitions

Advanced: 60 (30 per side) repetitions

How To Perform The Exercise

1. Begin standing straight up with your feet shoulder width apart.
2. Cross your arms in front of you and place the palm of your right hand over the back of your left hand. This is the starting position.
3. Raise your left arm straight out in front of you and then straight up overhead. Press your left arm as far back as possible.
4. Offer resistance with your right hand the whole way.
5. Breathe in as you raise your arms, exhale as you lower them.
6. Once you have completed the required repetitions repeat with your opposite arm.

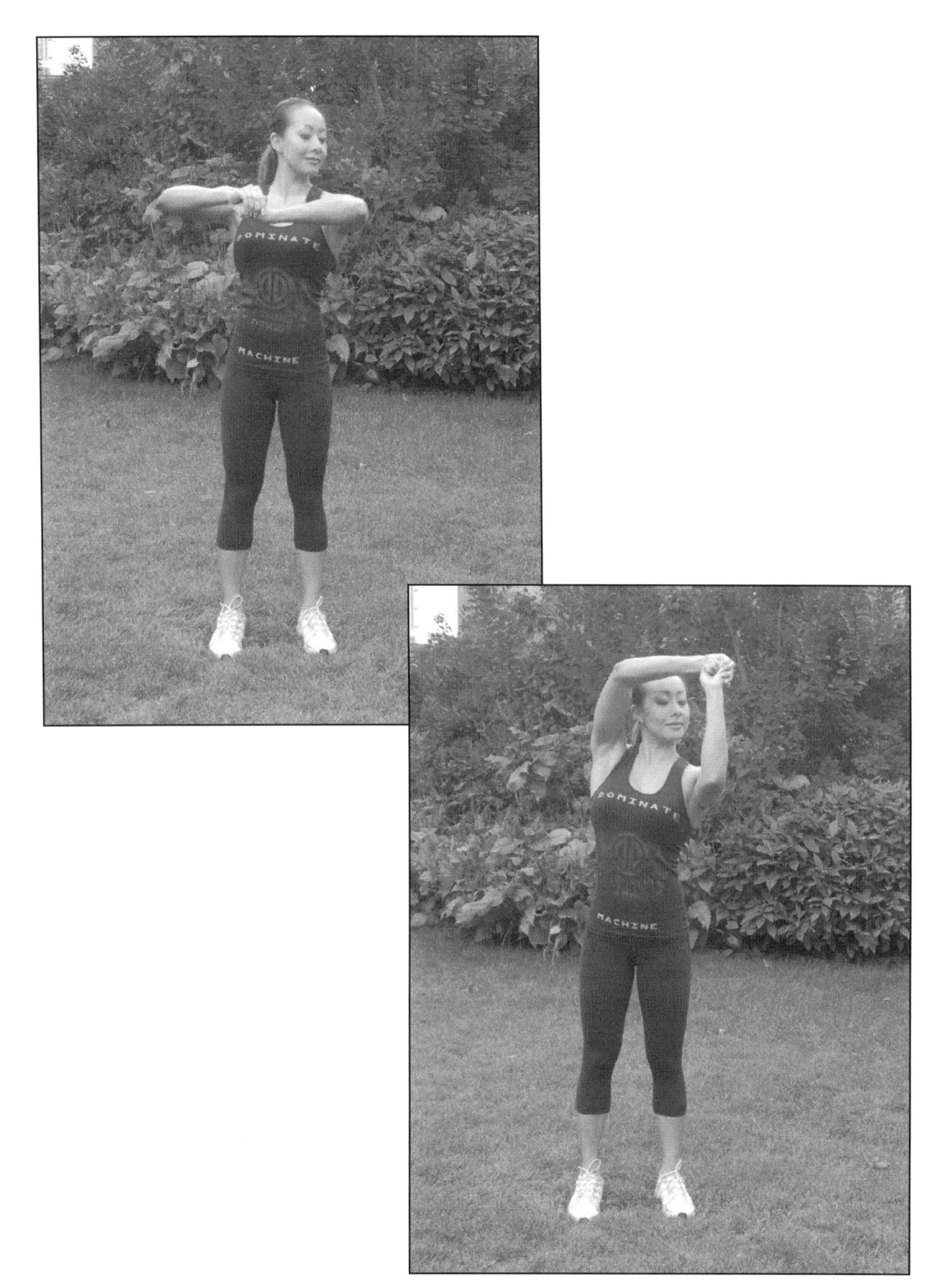

Shoulder Rotations

Number Of Repetitions

Beginner: 20 (10 per side) repetitions

Intermediate: 40 (20 per side) repetitions

Advanced: 60 (30 per side) repetitions

How To Perform The Exercise

1. Raise your right arm in front of you so that it is parallel to the floor.
2. Bend your right elbow at a 90 degree angle.
3. Place your left hand over the back of your right wrist. This is the starting position.
4. Rotate your right forearm up and away to your right as far as it will go.
5. Provide resistance with your left hand.
6. Once you have completed the required repetitions repeat with your opposite arm.

Exercises For The Back And Spine

Almost all of us suffer from back pain at one time or another. There are many reasons for, ranging from evolution to lifestyle, but really only one thing you can do about it, exercise and strengthen your back. The following exercises will do this for you, as well as give you a nice esthetic look.

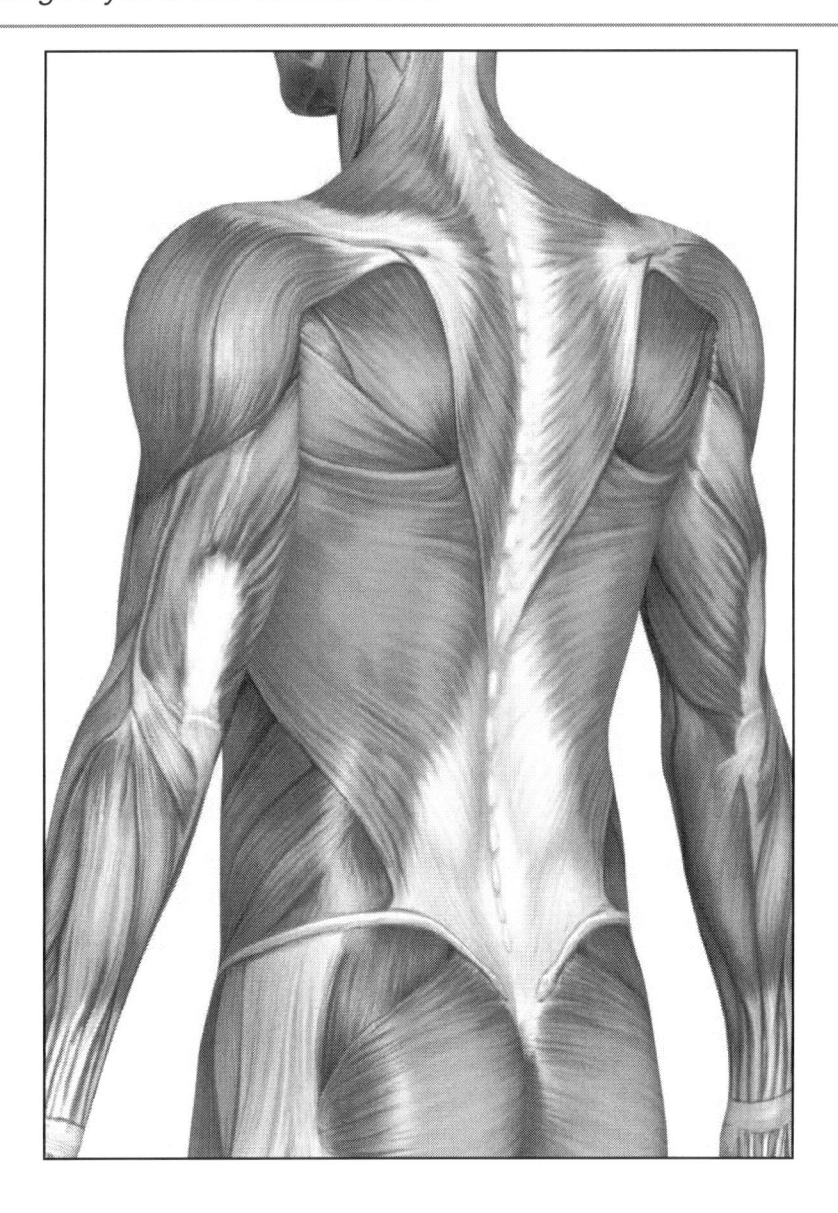

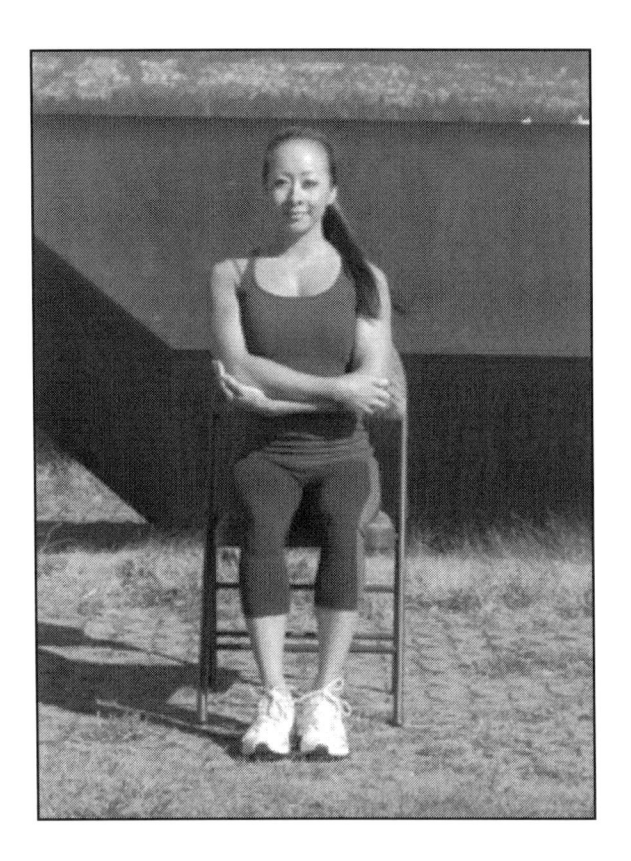

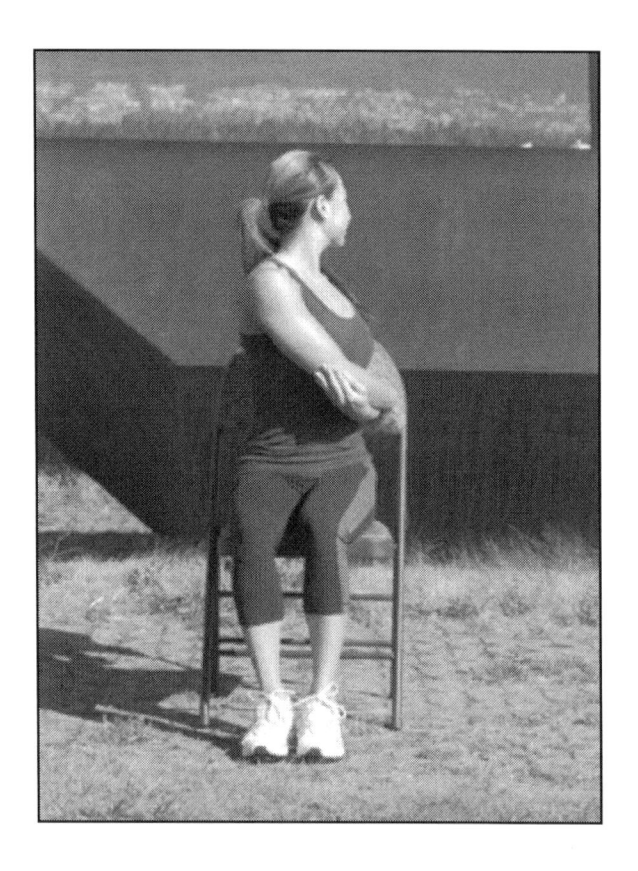

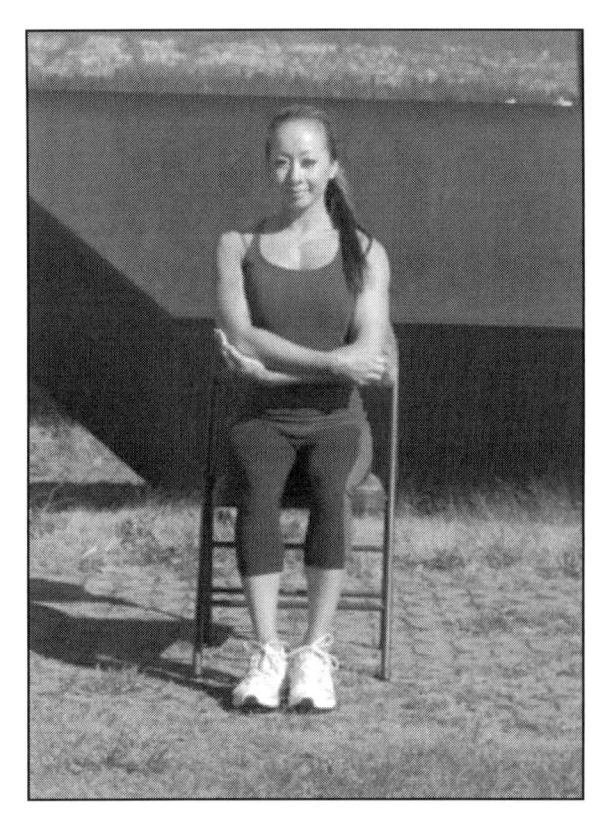

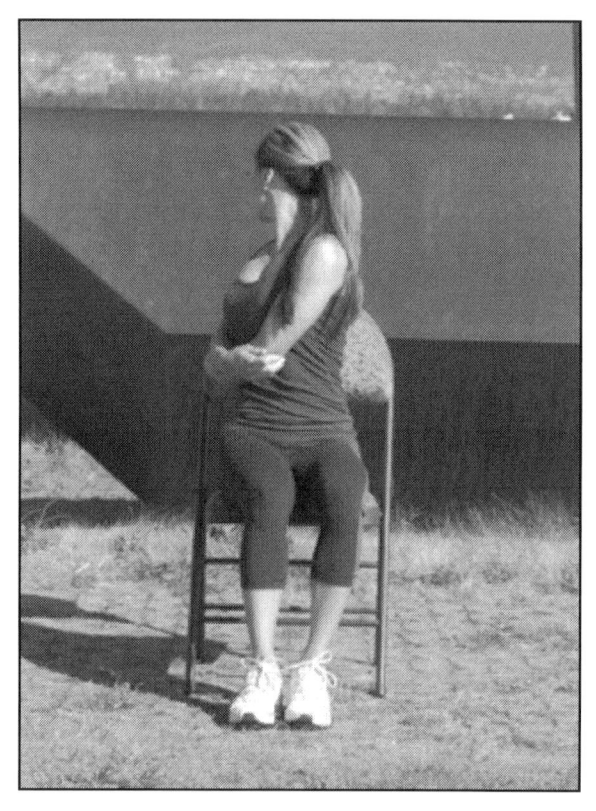

Copyright © 2010 David Nordmark. All rights reserved.
www.animal-kingdom-workouts.com

Page 76

Sitting Spine Twist

This exercise is excellent for loosening and strengthening the spine.

Number Of Repetitions

Beginner: 20 repetitions

Intermediate: 40 repetitions

Advanced: 60 repetitions

How To Perform The Exercise

1. Sit in a sturdy chair with your feet flat on the ground.
2. Cross your arms in front of you. This is the beginning position.
3. Turn your head and torso to the left. It's almost like you're trying to see something that is behind your left shoulder.
4. Return to the beginning position and then turn your head and torso to the right. This counts as one repetition.
5. Repeat until you have completed the required repetitions.

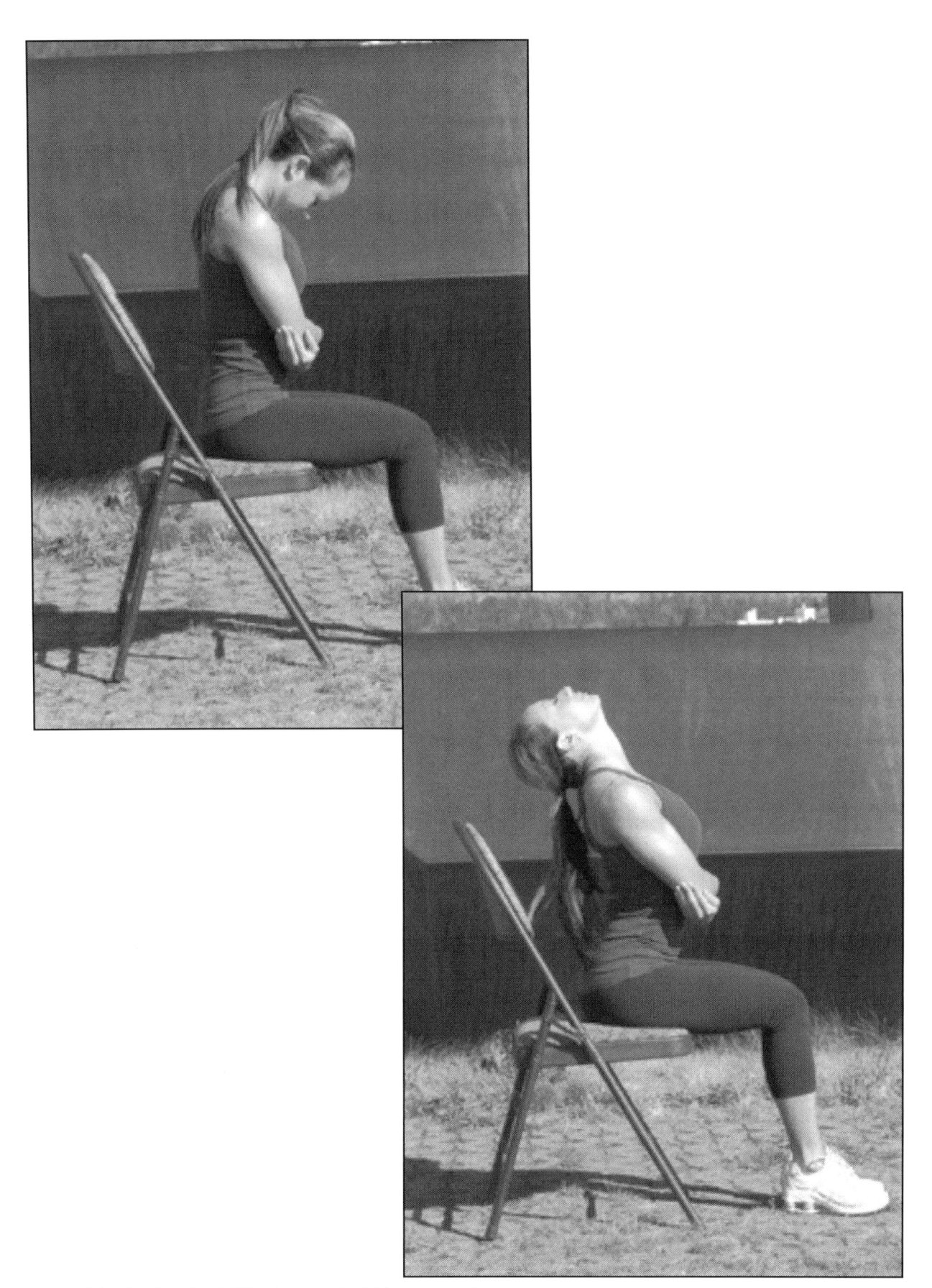

www.animal-kingdom-workouts.com

Page 78

Upper Spine Stretch

This simple movements loosens the top of the spine.

Number Of Repetitions

Beginner: 5 repetitions

Intermediate: 10 repetitions

Advanced: 20 repetitions

How To Perform The Exercise

1. Sit in a sturdy chair with your feet flat on the ground.
2. Cross your arms in front of you. This is the beginning position.
3. Keeping your back straight bend your neck forward so that your chin touches your chest.
4. Return your head to the beginning position and then bend your head backwards as far as you can.
5. One forward and one backward head movement constitutes one repetition.

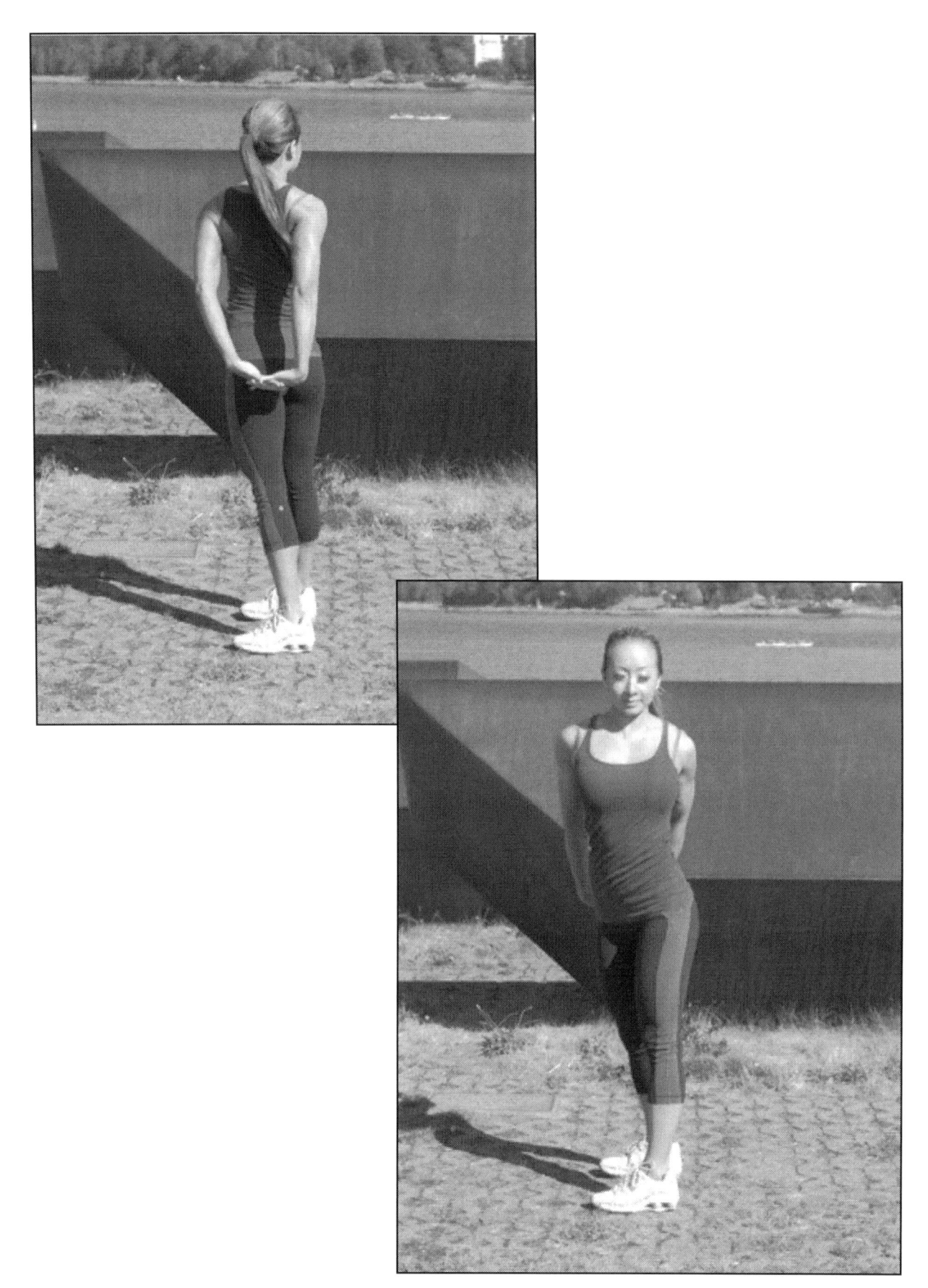

Copyright © 2010 David Nordmark. All rights reserved.
www.animal-kingdom-workouts.com

Standing Spine Twist

This exercise is essentially a variation of the sitting spine twist and is also excellent for keeping the spine limber.

Number Of Repetitions

Beginner: 5 repetitions

Intermediate: 10 repetitions

Advanced: 20 repetitions

How To Perform The Exercise

1. Stand with your legs straight and your feet shoulder width apart.
2. Clasp your hands behind your back with your arms straight. This is the beginning position.
3. Turn your upper body to the left while keeping your legs straight.
4. Return to the beginning position and then turn your body to the right.
5. One left to right motion constitutes one repetition.
6. Exhale as you twist to one side, inhale as your return to the neutral position.

Copyright © 2010 David Nordmark. All rights reserved.
www.animal-kingdom-workouts.com

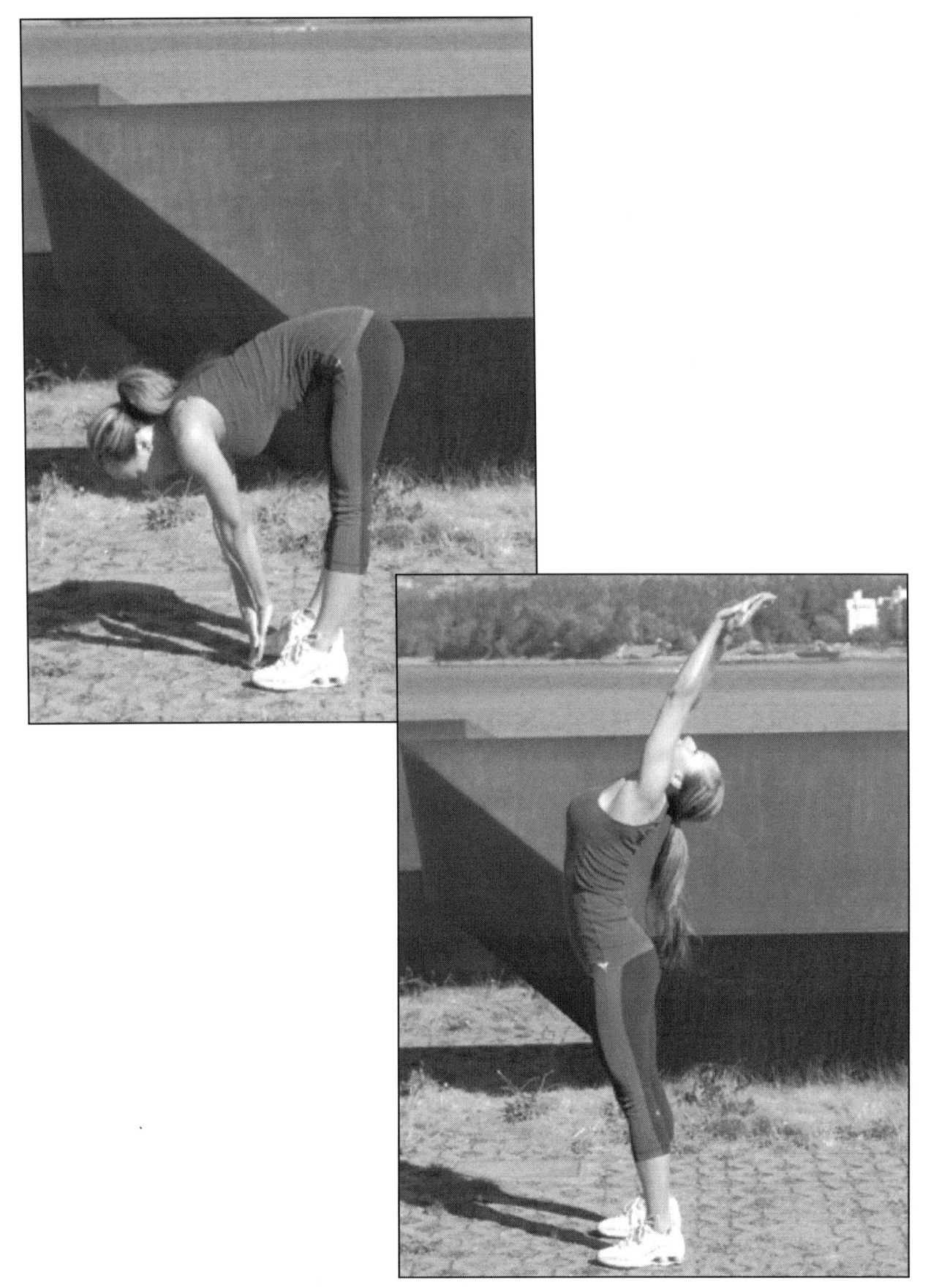

Standing Spine Bends

This exercise is essentially a variation of the sitting spine twist and is also excellent for keeping the spine limber.

Number Of Repetitions

Beginner: 10 repetitions

Intermediate: 20 repetitions

Advanced: 40 repetitions

How To Perform The Exercise

1. Stand with your feet shoulder width apart and your arms straight in front of you with one hand over the other.
2. Bend forward from the waist and touch your hand to the ground.
3. Stand straight up again while bringing your arms straight above your head. Now stretch backwards with your hands bending your lower back.
4. One forward and one backward bend constitutes one repetition.
5. Exhale during the forward bending motion, inhale as you bend backwards.
6. If you need to bend your knees to touch the ground feel free to do so.
7. Always keep your stomach muscles tight to protect your lower back.

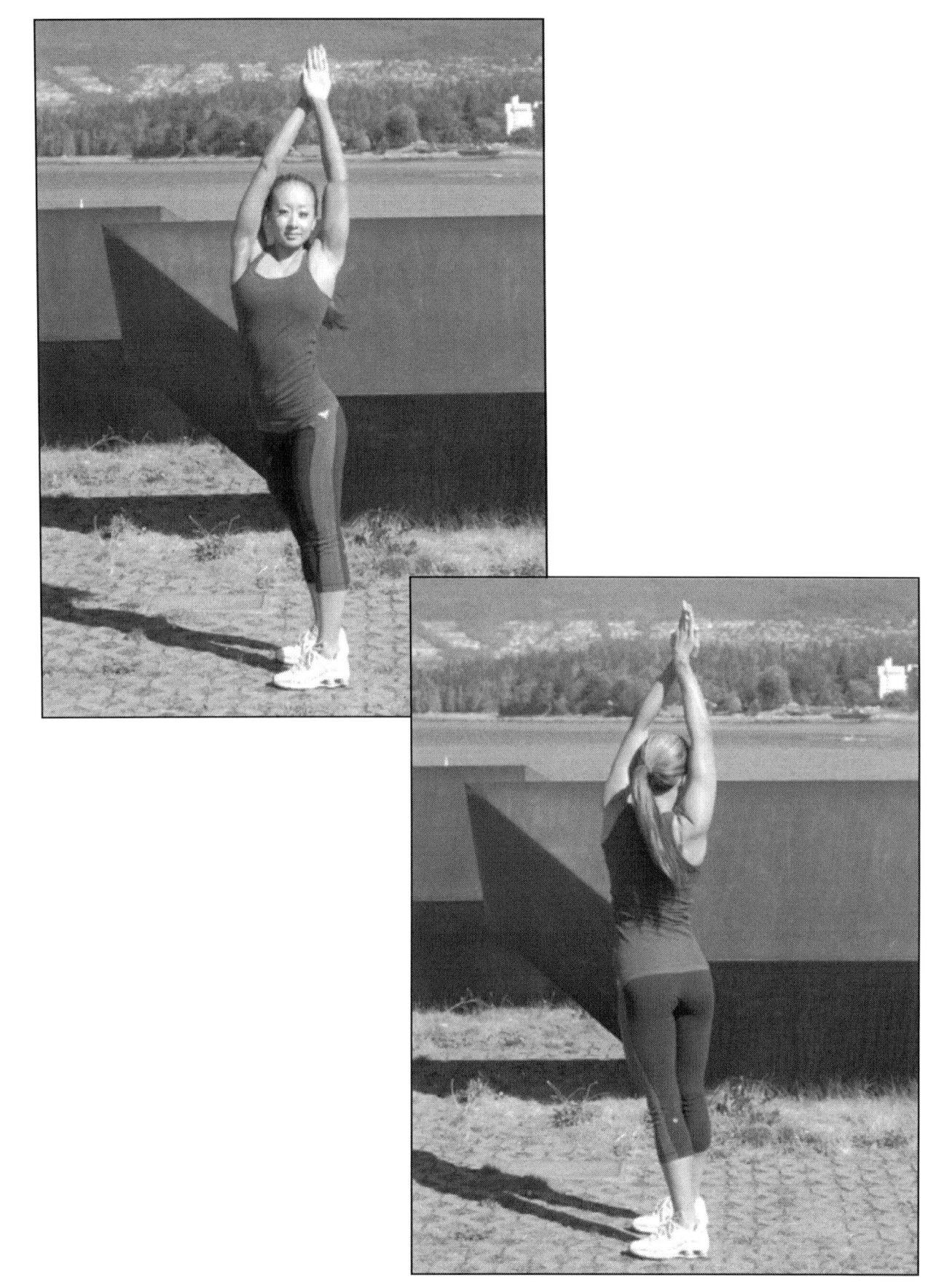

Copyright © 2010 David Nordmark. All rights reserved.
www.animal-kingdom-workouts.com

Spine Spirals

Number Of Repetitions

Beginner: 10 repetitions

Intermediate: 20 repetitions

Advanced: 40 repetitions

How To Perform The Exercise

1. Stand straight up with your feet together and your arms straight above your head.
2. Your hands should be crossed.
3. This is the beginning neutral position.
4. Turn your upper body to the left as much as possible, then turn to the right.
5. Exhale as you twist your body to one side, inhale as you return your body to the neutral position
6. One left right turn constitutes one repetition.

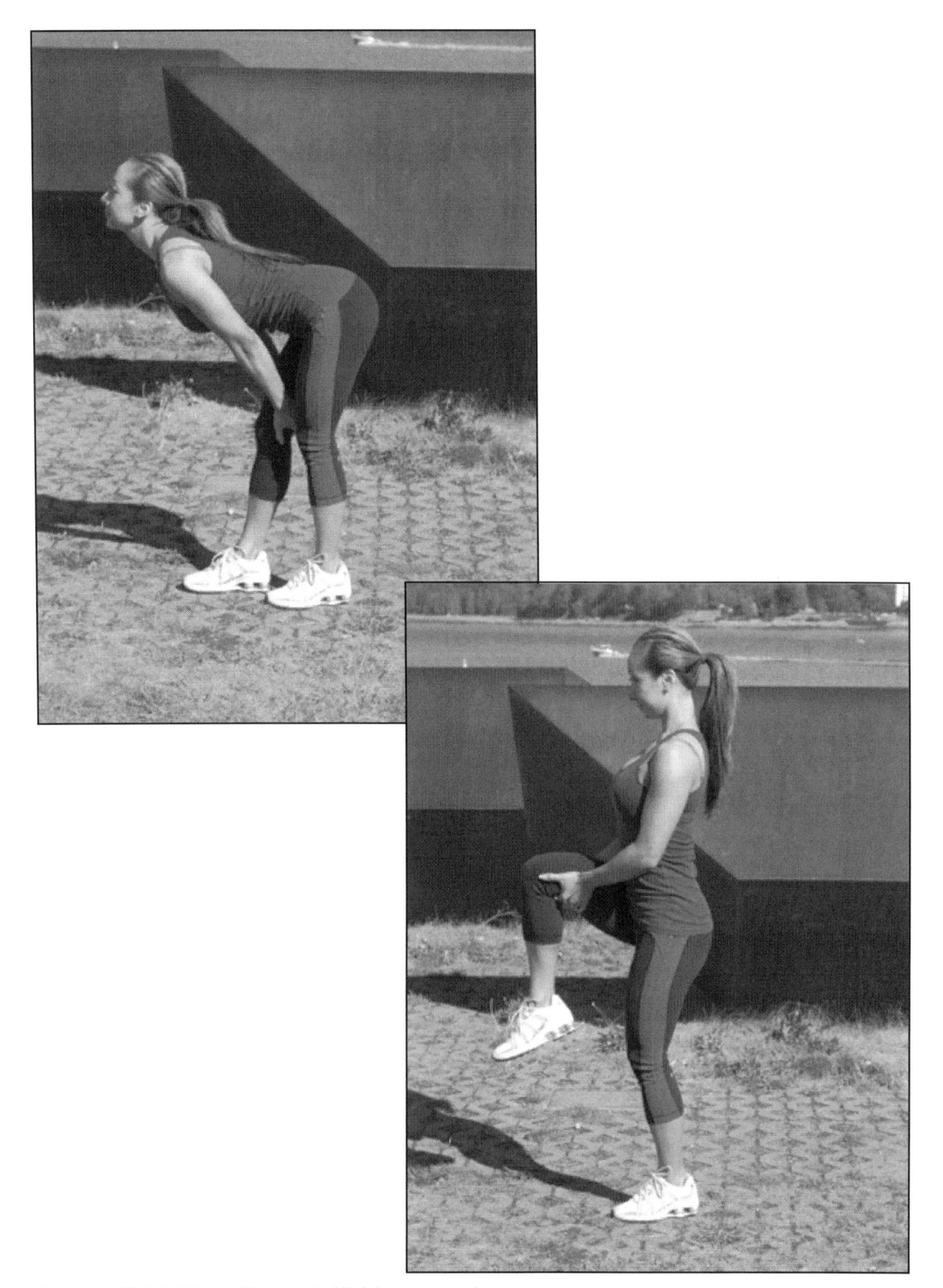

Isotonic Deadlift

This is an isotonic version of the deadlift that really works your latissimus dorsi muscles. It will also help you with your intramuscular coordination and balance. At first, this exercise will feel extremely awkward. When starting, it is best to take it easy and just get used to the movement. You can increase the resistance offered by your leg when you get more comfortable with the exercise.

Number Of Repetitions

Beginner: 10 (5 per leg) repetitions
Intermediate: 20 (10 per leg) repetitions
Advanced: 40 (20 per leg) repetitions

How To Perform The Exercise

1. Begin with your right leg slightly in front of your left leg.
2. Tightly clasp both hands behind the knee of the right leg.
3. Using your back muscles, attempt to stand up straight while resisting with your right leg.
4. Keep your stomach muscles tight and your back as straight as possible at all times.
5. Once you have completed the necessary repetitions with your right leg repeat with your left.
6. At first this exercise will feel quite awkward as it does require some balance. Keep at it and your balance will improve along with your back strength.

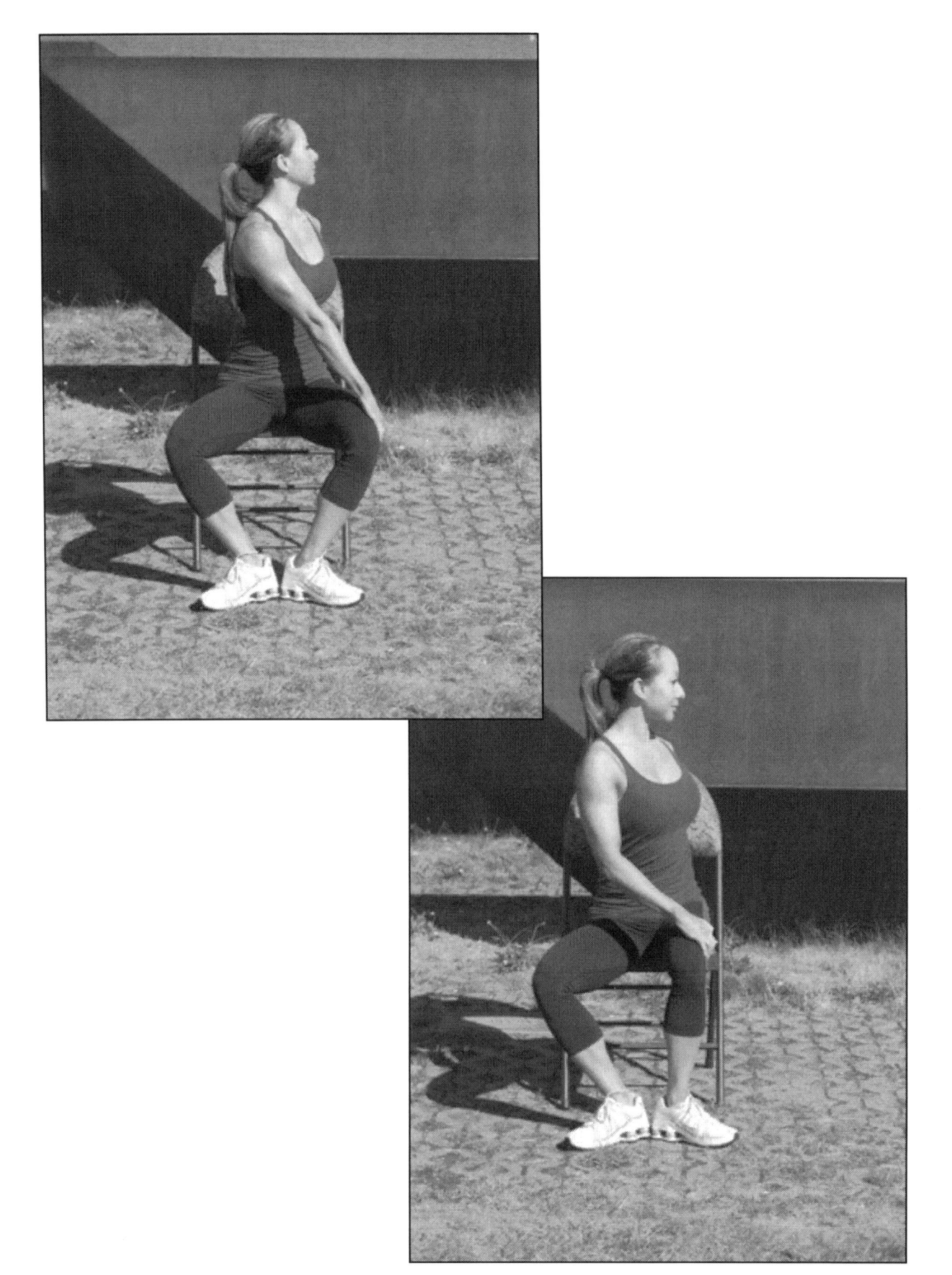

Sitting Back Pull

Like the isotonic deadlift, this exercise also works your latissimus dorsi muscles. However, it doesn't require the same level of balance, so you will probably find it easier to perform.

Number Of Repetitions

Beginner: 10 (5 per leg) repetitions
Intermediate: 20 (10 per leg) repetitions
Advanced: 40 (20 per leg) repetitions

How To Perform The Exercise

1. Sit on the edge of a chair.
2. Put your feet together while spreading your knees apart.
3. Turn your torso to the right and place the palm of your left hand over the outside of your right knee.
4. Use your back muscles to pull your right knee while your right leg offers resistance.
5. Complete the necessary number of repetitions then switch legs.

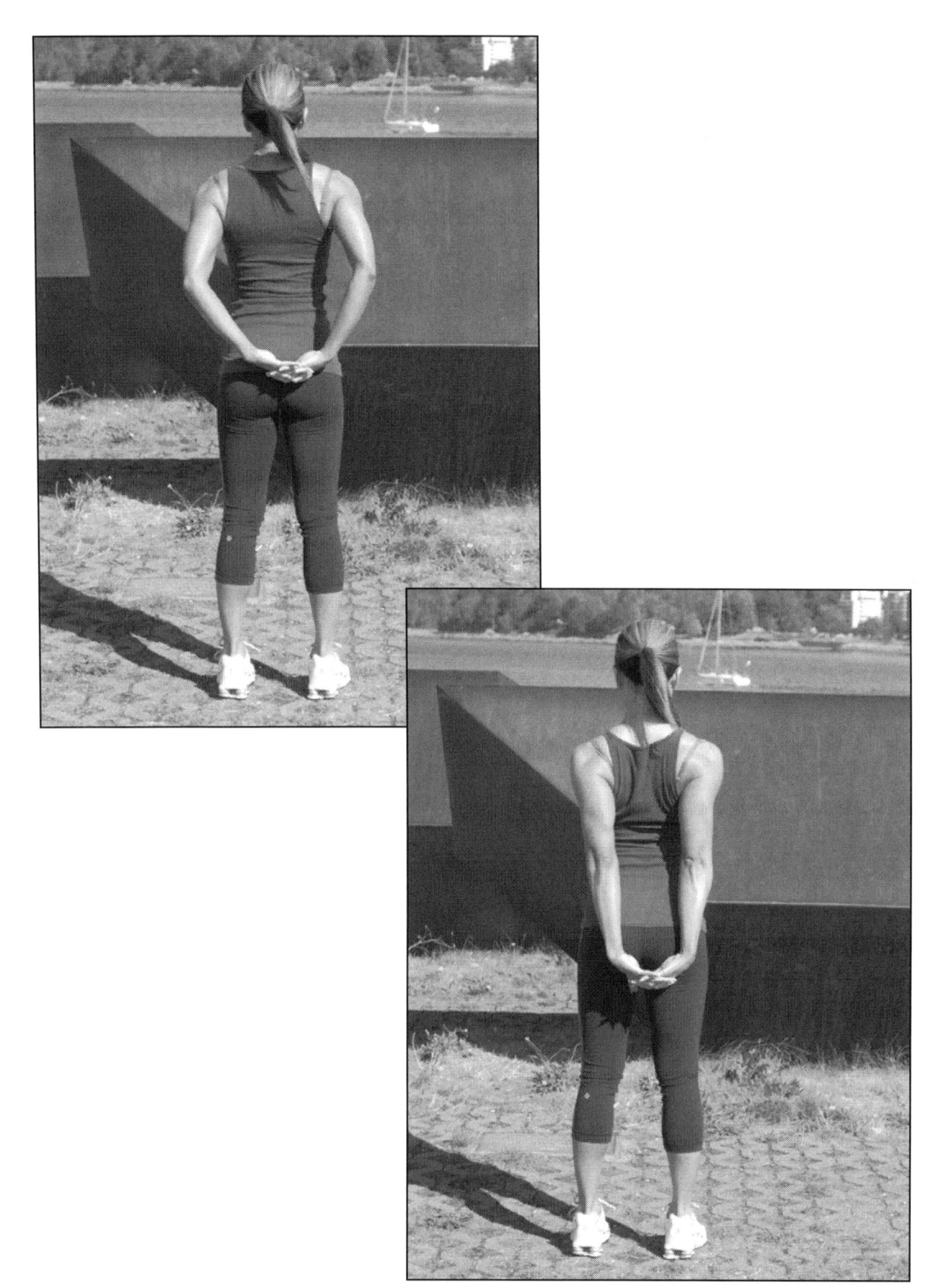

Shoulder Blade Contraction

This exercise will really hit the trapezius muscles, which extend from the base of the neck to the top of the shoulders through the middle of the back. Well developed trapezius muscles will help keep your neck strong and enhance your posture by preventing your shoulders from slouching.

Number Of Repetitions

Beginner: 5 repetitions
Intermediate: 20 repetitions
Advanced: 20 repetitions

How To Perform The Exercise

1. Begin standing with your feet shoulder width apart and your arms by your sides.
2. Clasp your hands firmly behind your back.
3. Pull your hands downwards while you bring your shoulder blades together and downwards.
4. Relax your shoulder blades and allow your hands to come up. This constitutes a single repetition.

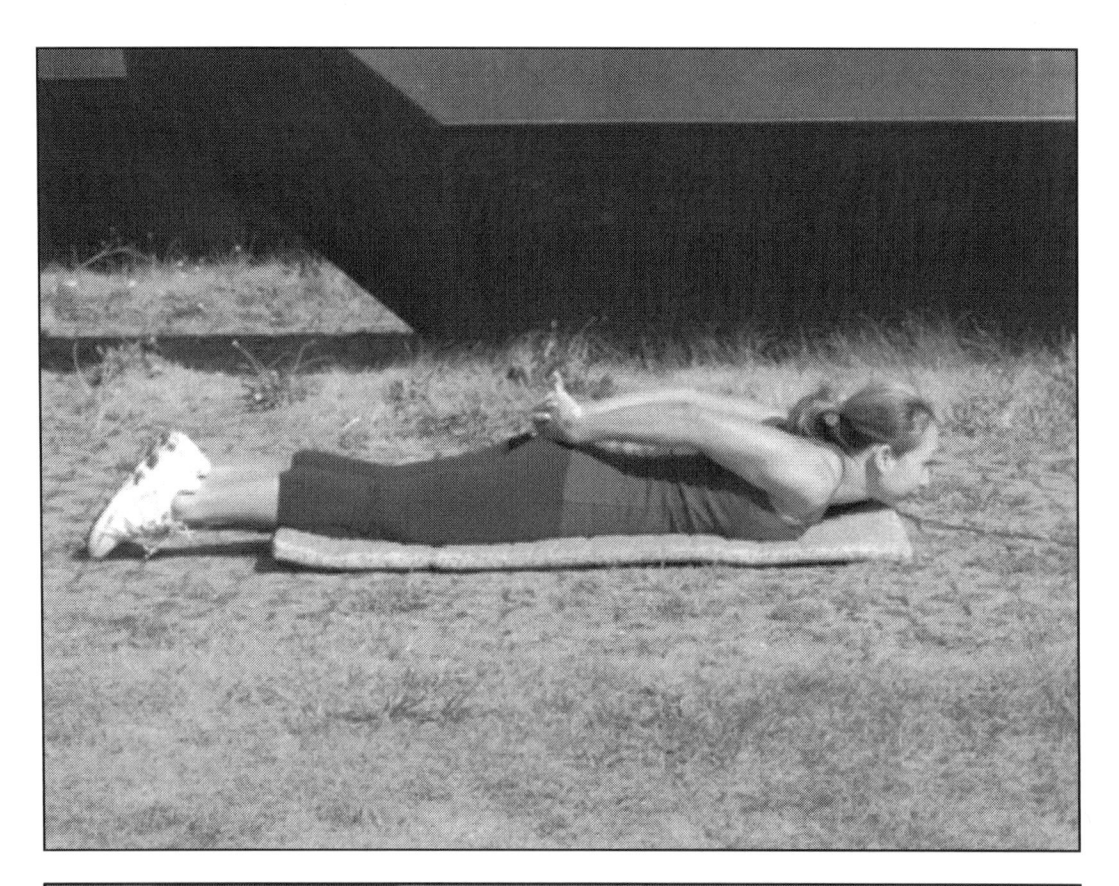

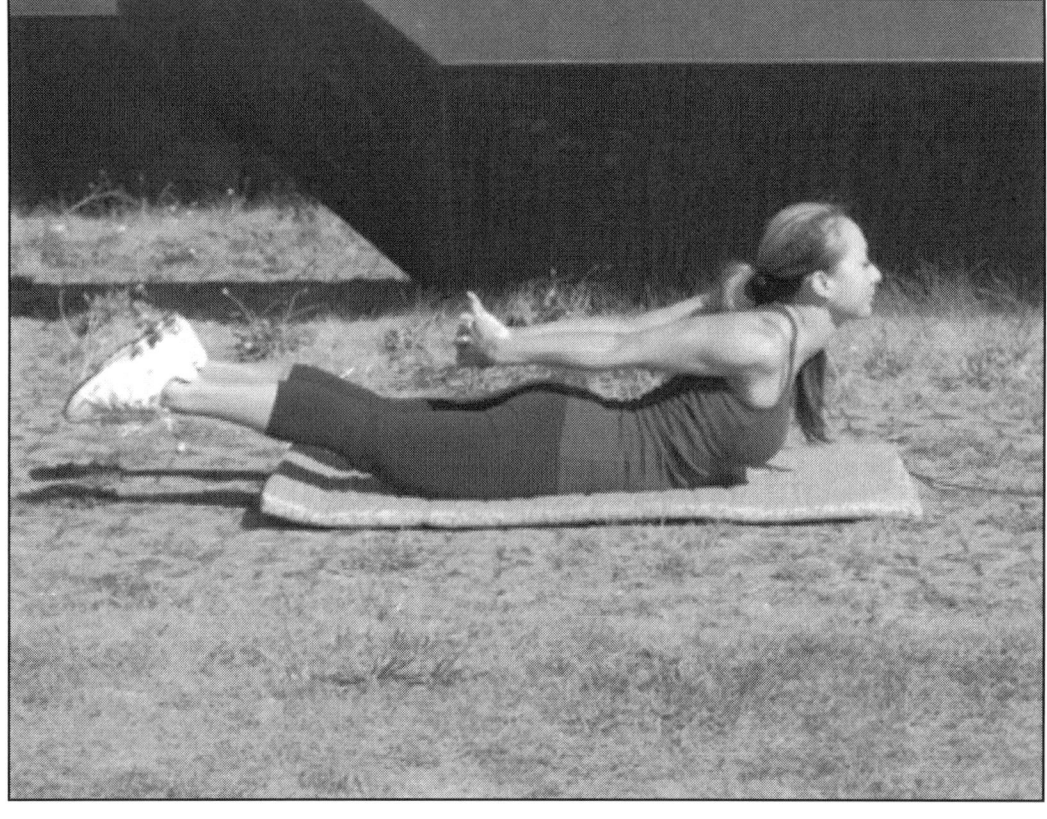

Back Flex

Exercises that allow you to bend your back backwards are incredibly important in order to keep your spine youthful and supple. This is exactly what the Back Flex does.

Number Of Repetitions

Beginner: 5 repetitions

Intermediate: 10 repetitions

Advanced: 15 repetitions

How To Perform The Exercise

1. Lie flat on the ground with your chest facing the floor.
2. Clasp your hands behind you.
3. Pull your hands backwards while your simultaneously raise your feet off the ground. This should result in only your stomach being on the ground.
4. When you perform this exercise flex your butt muscles to protect your lower spine.

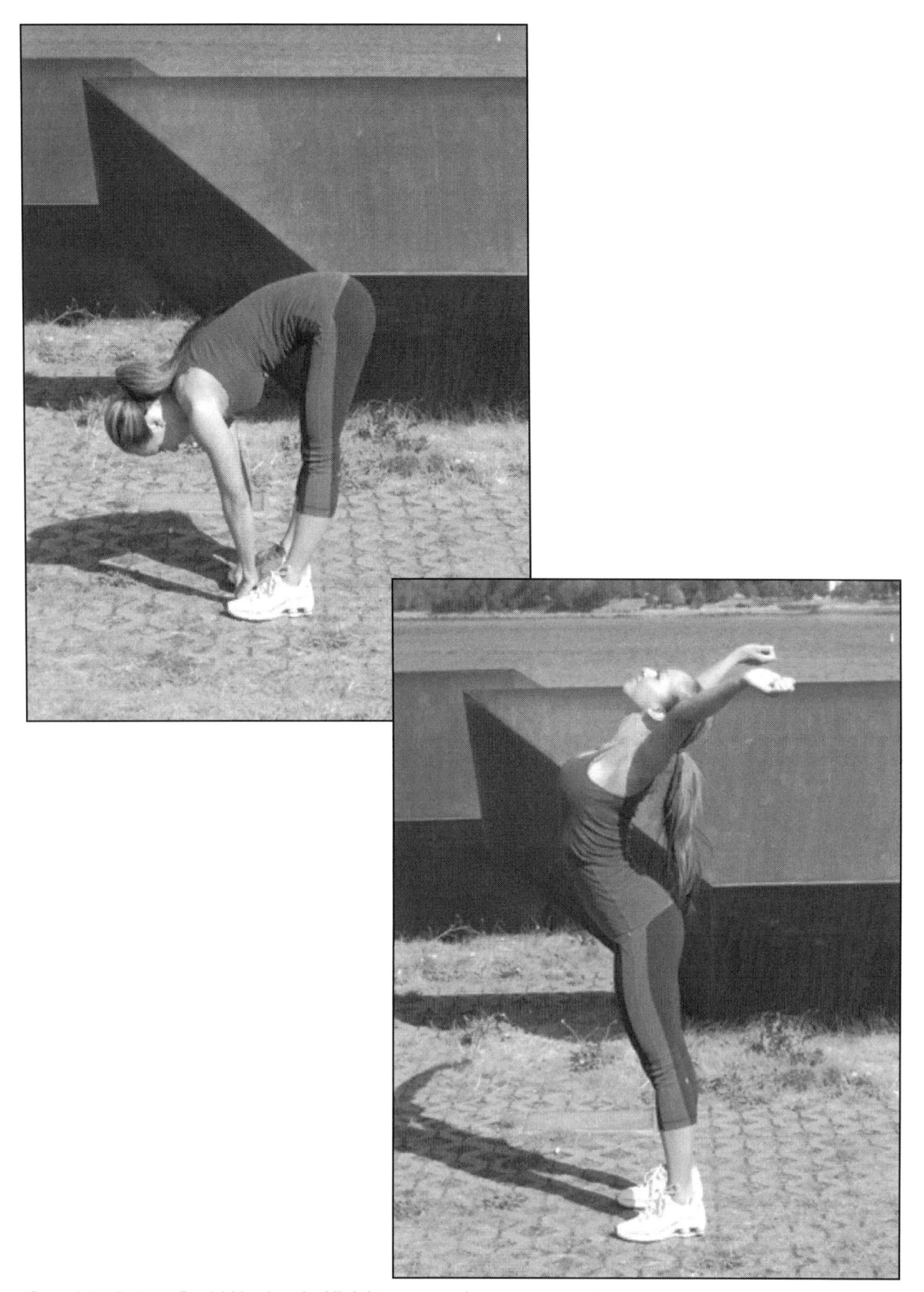

Standing Back Flex

This exercise will develop your back muscles while keeping your spine healthy at the same time.

Number Of Repetitions

Beginner: 5 repetitions

Intermediate: 10 repetitions

Advanced: 15 repetitions

How To Perform The Exercise

1. Begin by standing with your feet shoulder width apart with your hands by your sides.
2. Bend forward at the waist and place your hands on the floor in front of you. You can bend your knees if you need to.
3. Stand straight up again and then bend backwards so that you are looking at the ceiling. As you do so, stretch your arms as far as you can to the sides while make a fist with your hands. You should really feel the stretch in your chest muscles as you do this.
4. One forward bend and backward bend constitutes one repetition.
5. Make sure you keep you stomach muscles tight to protect your lower back.
6. Exhale as you bend forward, inhale as you bend backwards.

Arm Exercises

Other than flat abdominals nothing quite says "I'm healthy" than well developed triceps and biceps. Aside from appearance, strong arms can also enhance your athletic performance in any sport your play. Although most people focus on the biceps, developing the triceps is equally important. The following exercises do both.

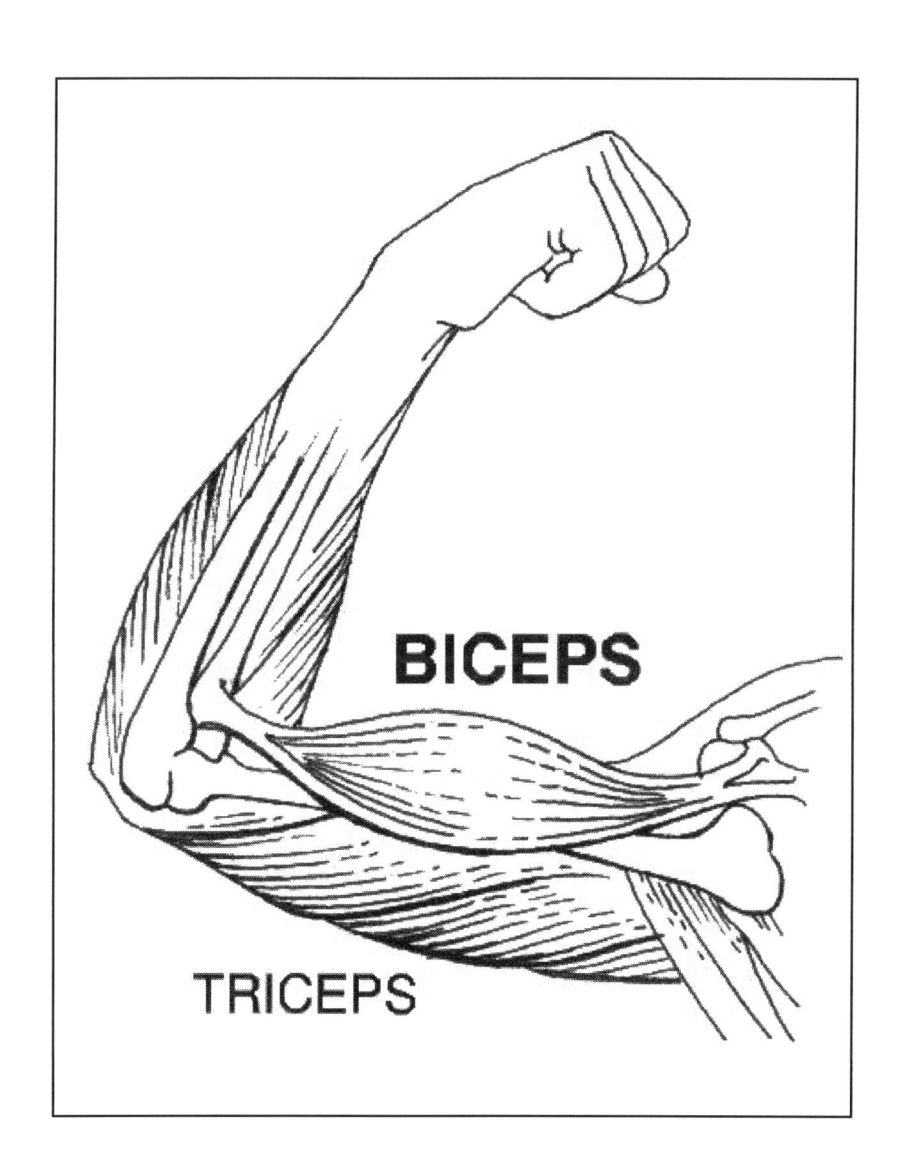

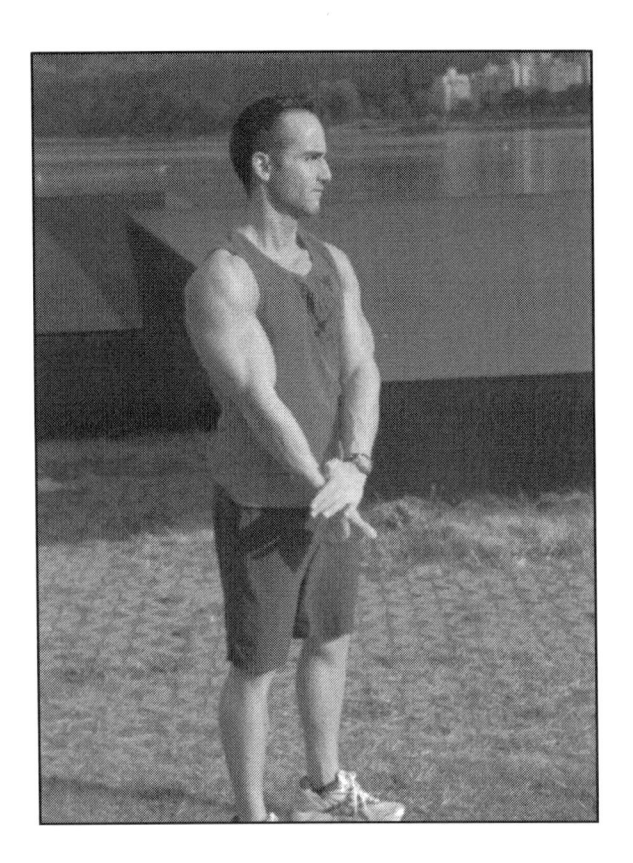

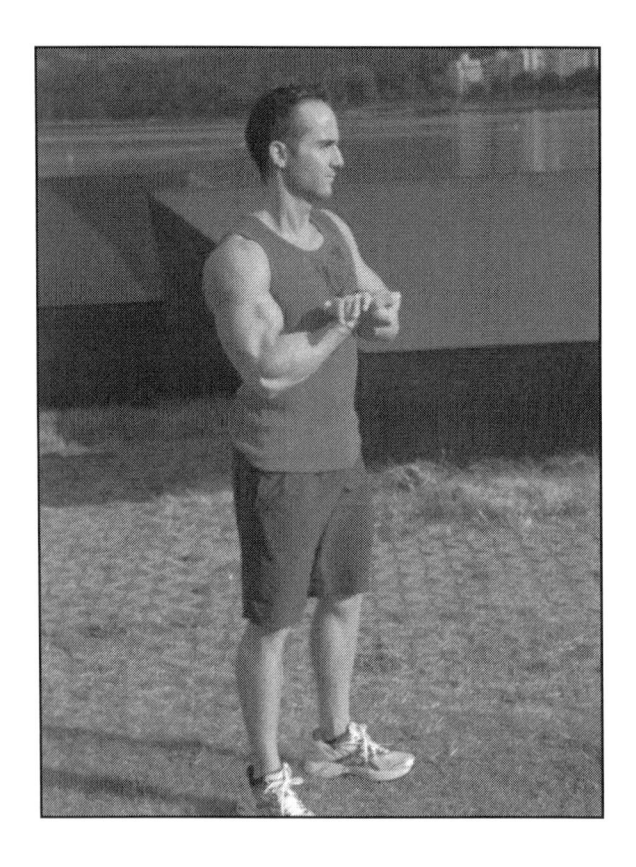

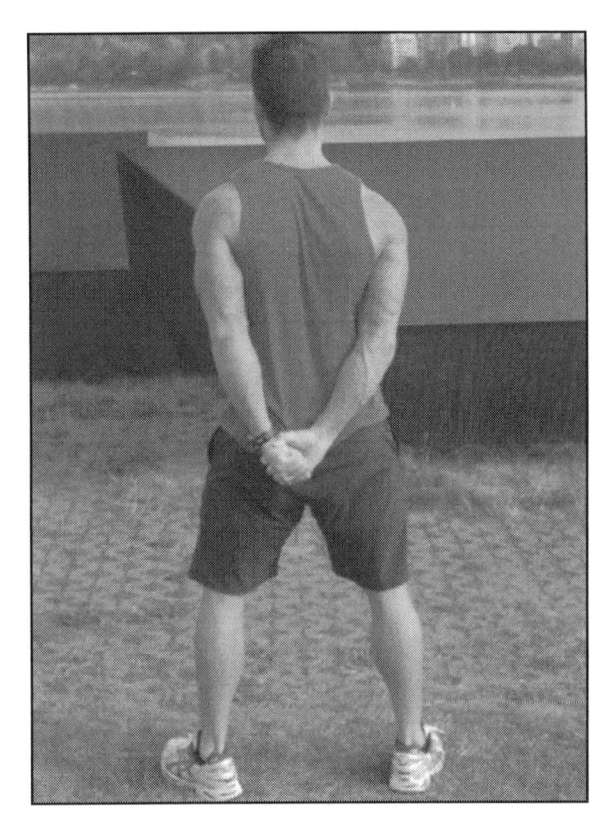

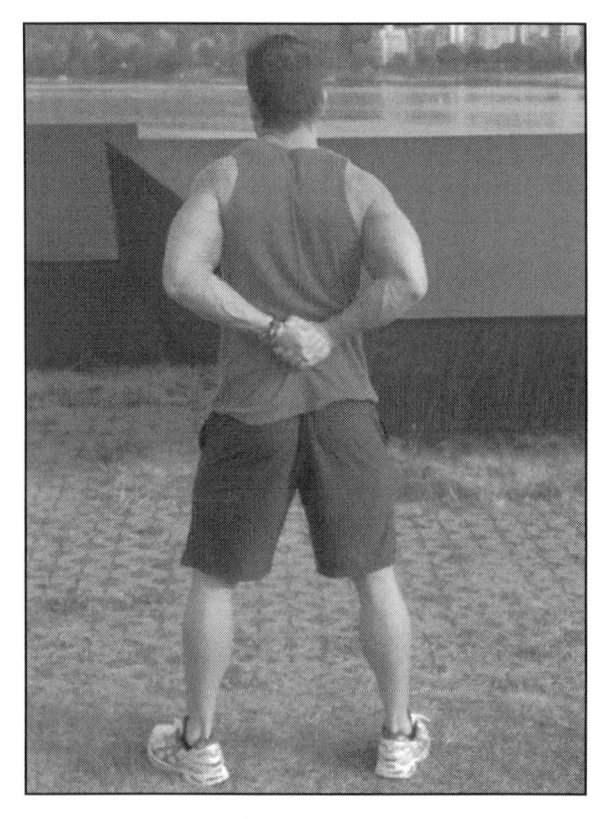

Biceps Curls

This exercise will help you build and define your biceps.

Number Of Repetitions

Beginner: 20 (5 in front, 5 in back then switch arms) repetitions

Intermediate: 40 (10 in front, 10 in back then switch arms) repetitions

Advanced: 60 (15 in front, 15 in back then switch arms) repetitions

How To Perform The Exercise

1. Begin standing straight up with your feet shoulder width apart.
2. Bend your right arm so that your right palm is facing upwards in front of your body.
3. Place your left hand over your right wrist.
4. Curl your right hand up, resisting with your left hand.
5. Now put your right arm behind your back with your palm facing upwards.
6. Place your left hand over your right wrist.
7. Curl your right hand up, resisting with your left hand.
8. Once your have completed 5 in the front and 5 in the back switch to work your left arm.

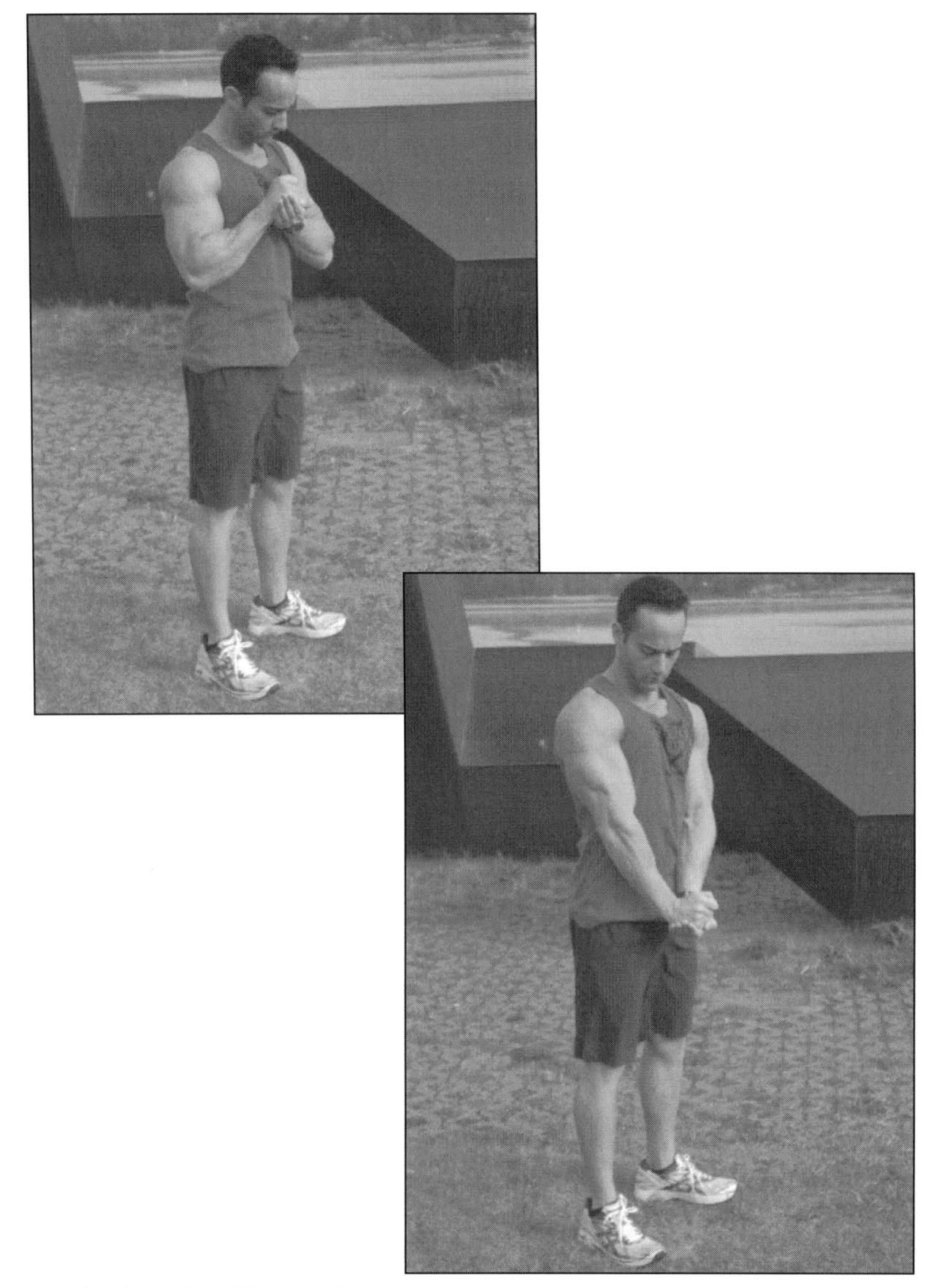

Triceps Press Down

This exercise will help you build and define your triceps.

Number Of Repetitions

Beginner: 20 (10 per side) repetitions

Intermediate: 40 (20 per side) repetitions

Advanced: 60 (30 per side) repetitions

How To Perform The Exercise

1. Begin standing with your feet shoulder width apart.
2. Bend your right arm so that your right hand is almost at your shoulder.
3. Make a fist with your right hand and place your left hand below it. This is the starting position.
4. Force your right arm downwards, resisting with your left hand.
5. Return your right arm to the starting position and repeat.
6. Once your have completed the necessary repetitions, repeat with the opposite arm.

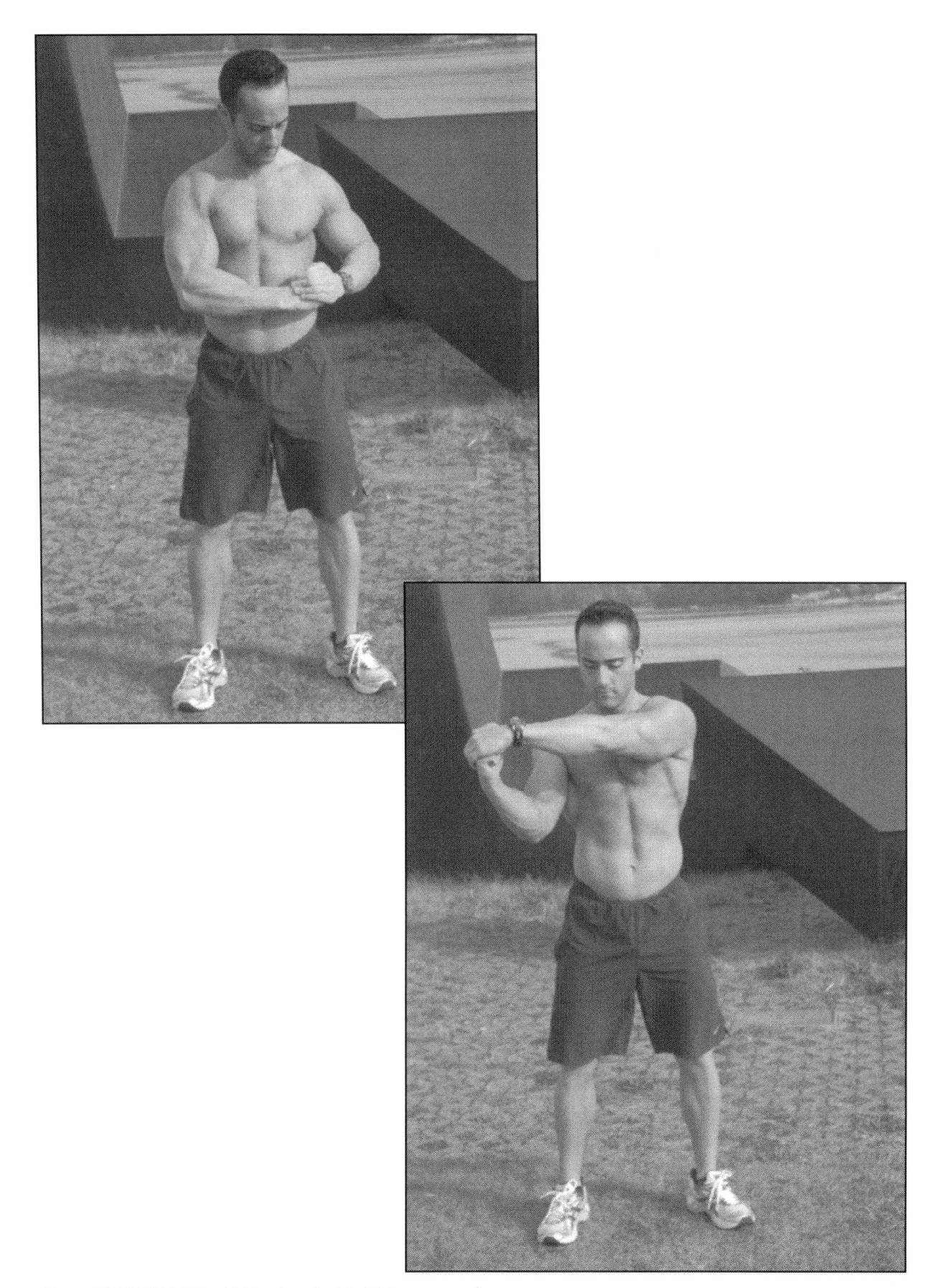

Copyright © 2010 David Nordmark. All rights reserved.
www.animal-kingdom-workouts.com

Page 102

Arm Rotations

This exercise will greatly aid your upper arm in gaining definition.

Number Of Repetitions

Beginner: 10 (5 per side) repetitions

Intermediate: 20 (10 per side) repetitions

Advanced: 40 (20 per side) repetitions

How To Perform The Exercise

1. Begin standing with your feet shoulder width apart.
2. Bend your right arm so that your right hand is by the left side of your waist.
3. Make a fist with your right hand.
4. Place your left hand over your right wrist. This is the starting position.
5. Resisting with your left hand, rotate your right arm from the shoulder to the right. You should feel this along your upper arm.
6. Strive to keep the 90 degree angle at your right elbow at all times.
7. Return your right arm to the starting position and repeat.
8. Once your have completed the necessary repetitions, repeat with the opposite arm.

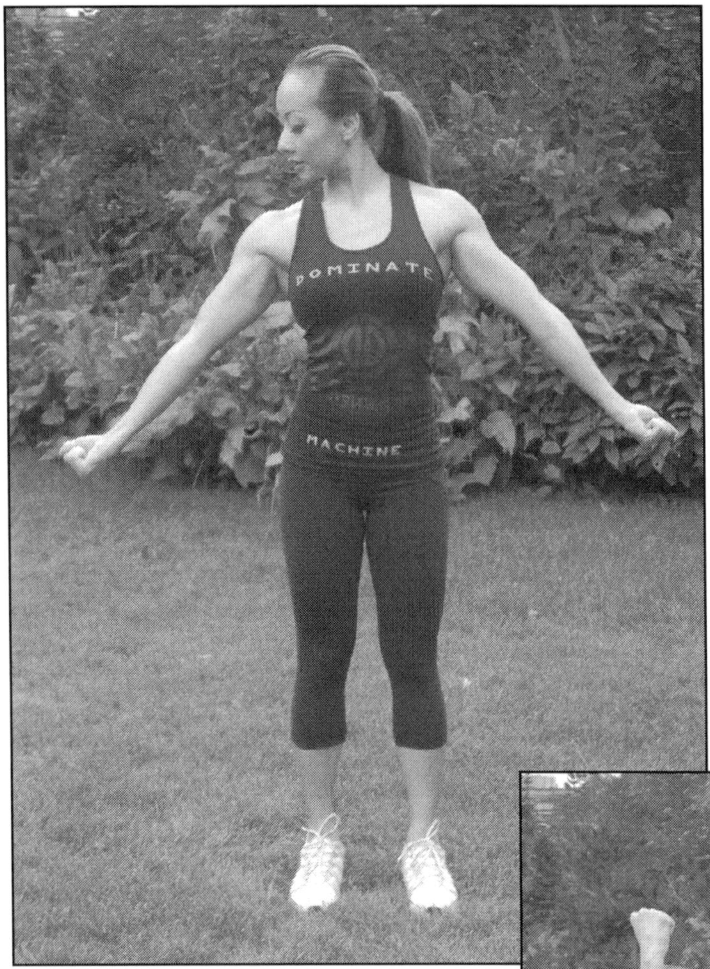
DOMINATE
MACHINE

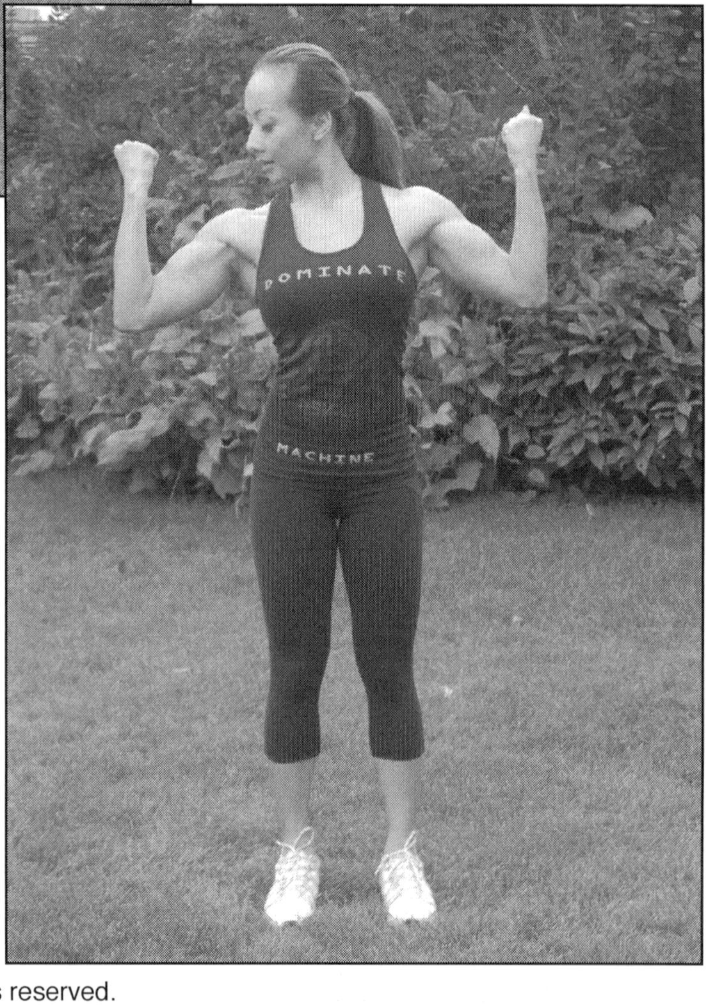
DOMINATE
MACHINE

Concentration Curls

This exercise develops both your biceps and triceps at the same time.

Number Of Repetitions

Beginner: 5 repetitions

Intermediate: 10 repetitions

Advanced: 20 repetitions

How To Perform The Exercise

1. Begin standing with your feet shoulder width apart and your arms by your sides.
2. Make a fist with both of your hands and rotate both of your arms inwards.
3. Curl both of your arms upwards while turning your wrists outwards.
4. As you lower your arms rotate your wrists inwards again.
5. You should be flexing your arms muscles constantly throughout this movement.

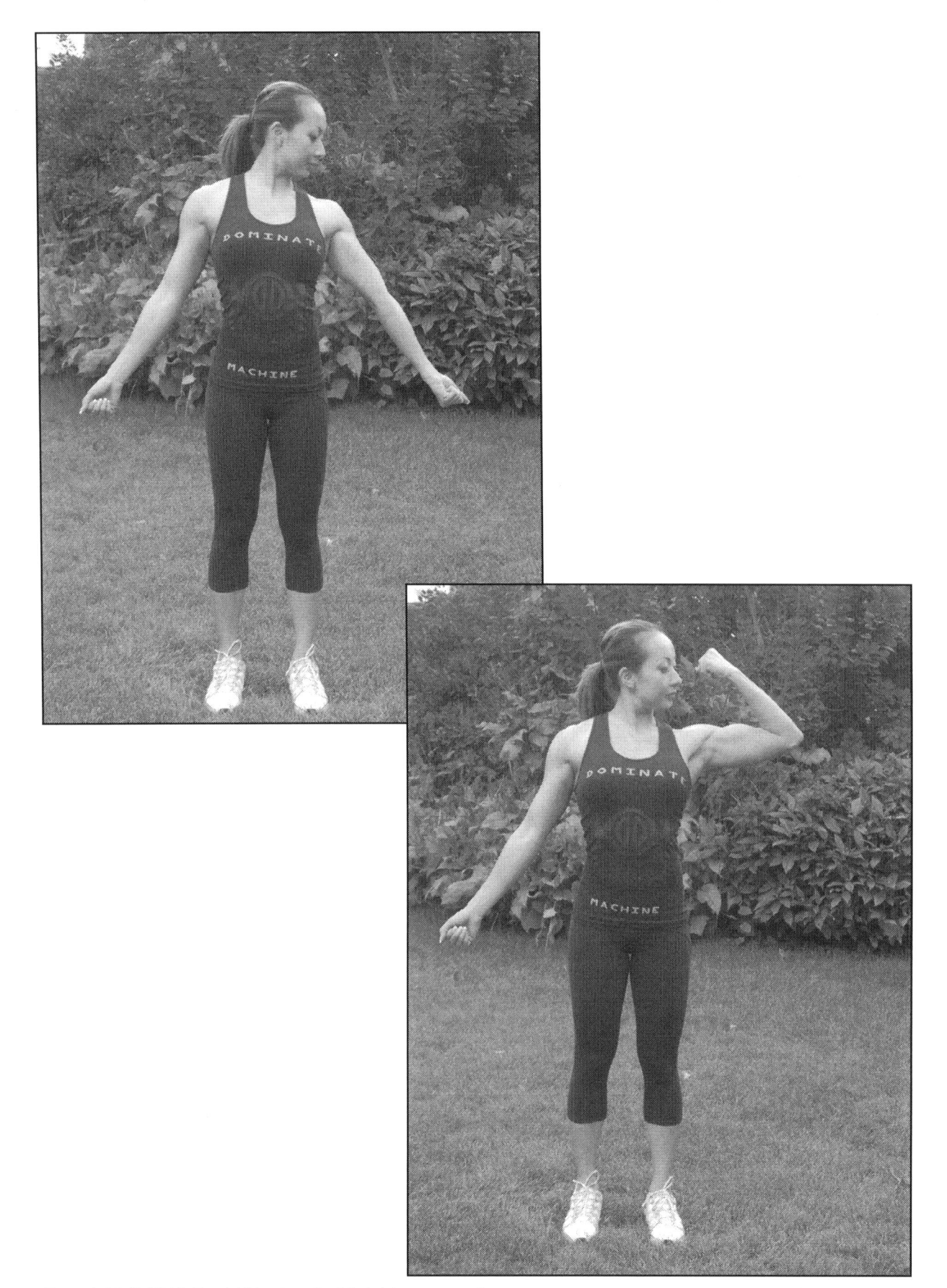

Concentration Flexes

When performing this exercise really focus on flexing your muscles to gain the maximum benefit.

Number Of Repetitions

Beginner: 10 (5 per side) repetitions

Intermediate: 20 (10 per side) repetitions

Advanced: 30 (15 per side) repetitions

How To Perform The Exercise

1. Begin standing with your feet shoulder width apart and your arms by your sides.
2. Make a fist with both of your hands and rotate both of your arms inwards.
3. Curl your right arm upwards while turning your wrists outwards.
4. As your lower your arm, rotate your wrists inwards again.
5. Repeat with the opposite arm.
6. You should be flexing your arms muscles constantly throughout this movement.

Leg Exercises

The hip and thigh muscles are the largest in the body. Athletic, muscular legs are not only attractive and vital to playing sports, but they are also one of the keys to staying young. "Healthy legs act like a heart for the lower body", someone once said, and they're right. If you want to stay young, you need to keep that blood pumping. Healthy legs will keep you young, strong and vital for life.

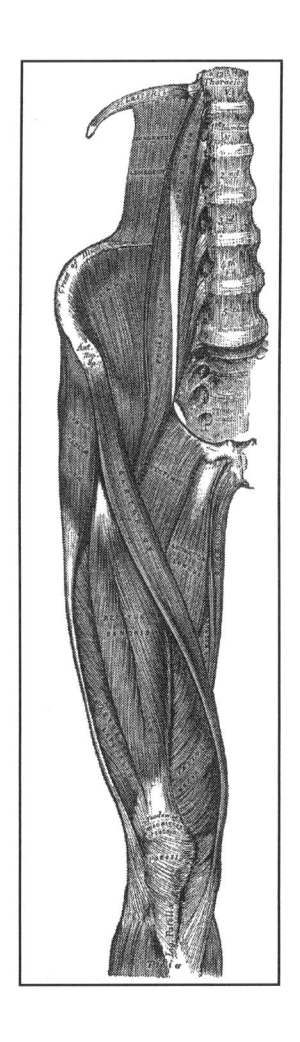

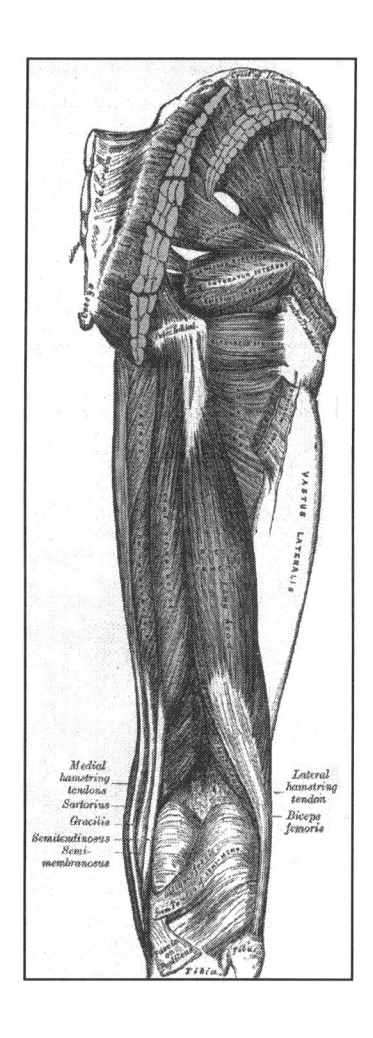

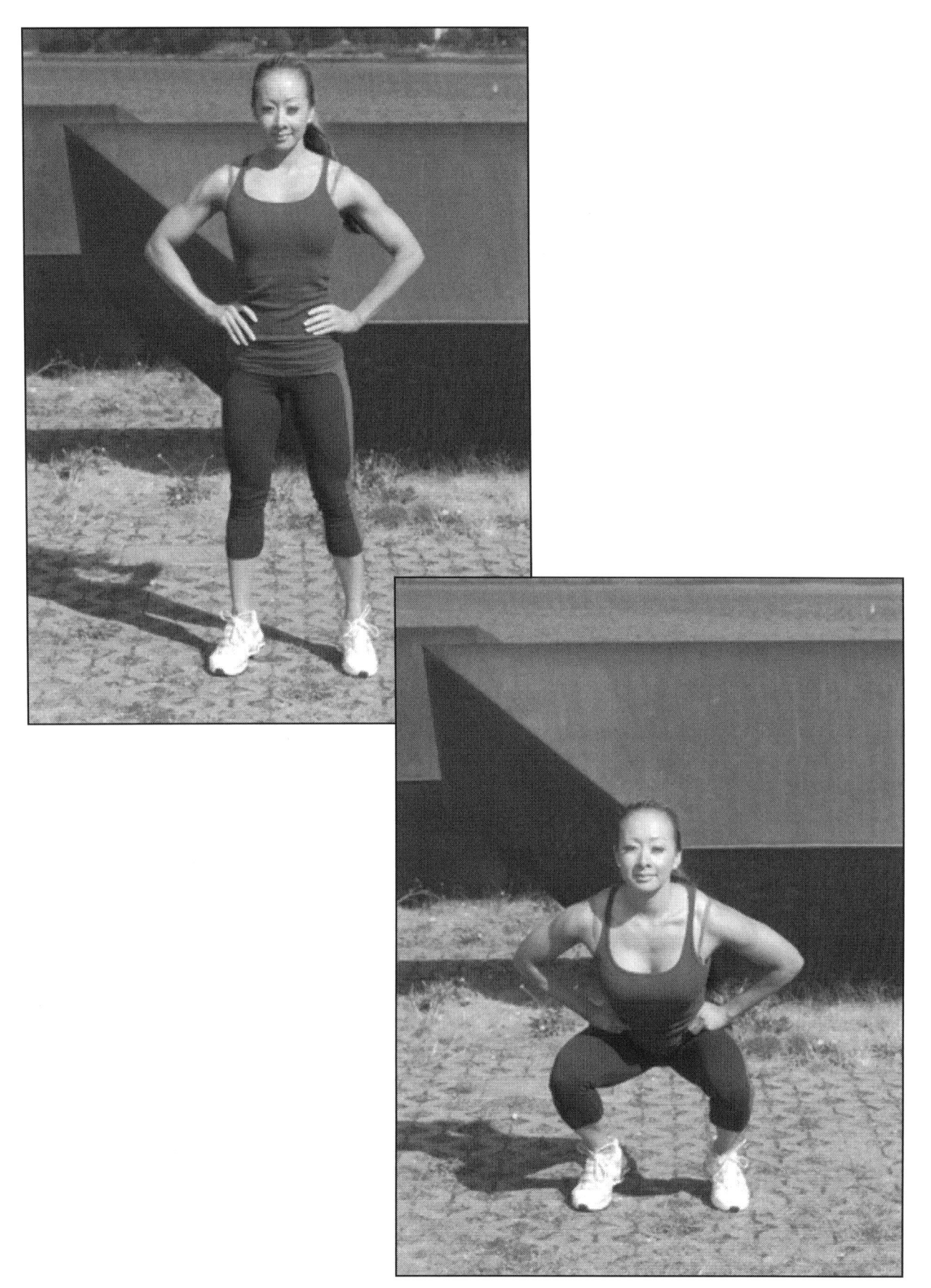

Frog Squats

This exercise will develop all of the muscles in your legs and improve your balance at the same time.

Number Of Repetitions

Beginner: 20 repetitions

Intermediate: 50 repetitions

Advanced: 100 repetitions

How To Perform The Exercise

1. Stand straight up with your feet slightly spread out in a V shape.
2. Place your hands on your hips and come up on your toes so that your heals are slightly off the ground.
3. Keeping your back straight, bend your knees so that you squat down and then press up again.
4. Exhale as you squat down, inhale as you come up.
5. Try to squat down far enough so that your thighs are parallel to the ground.

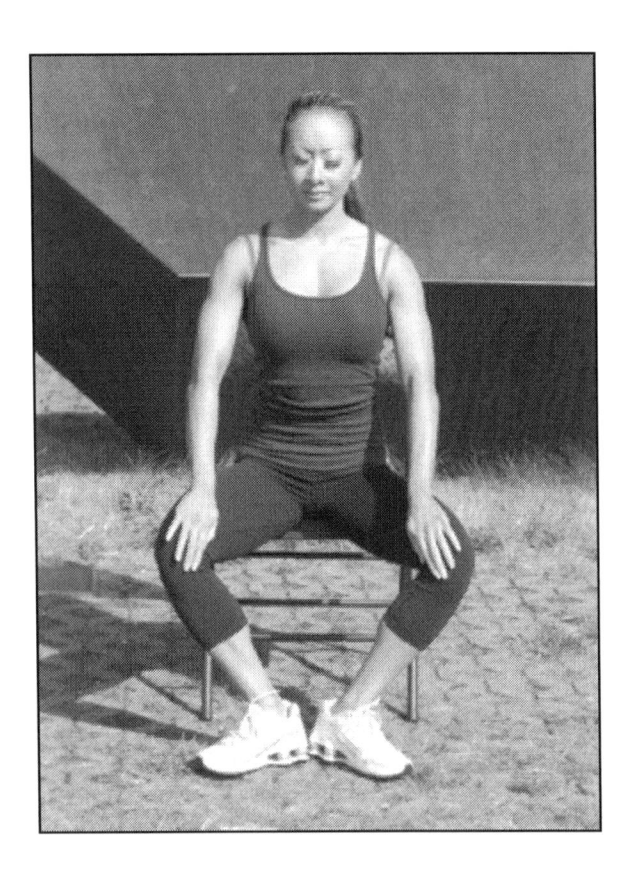

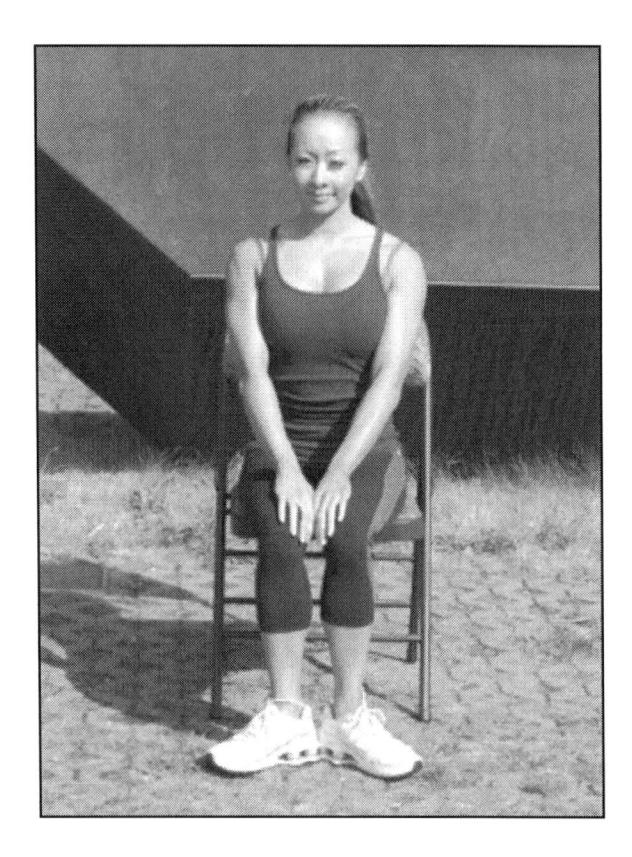

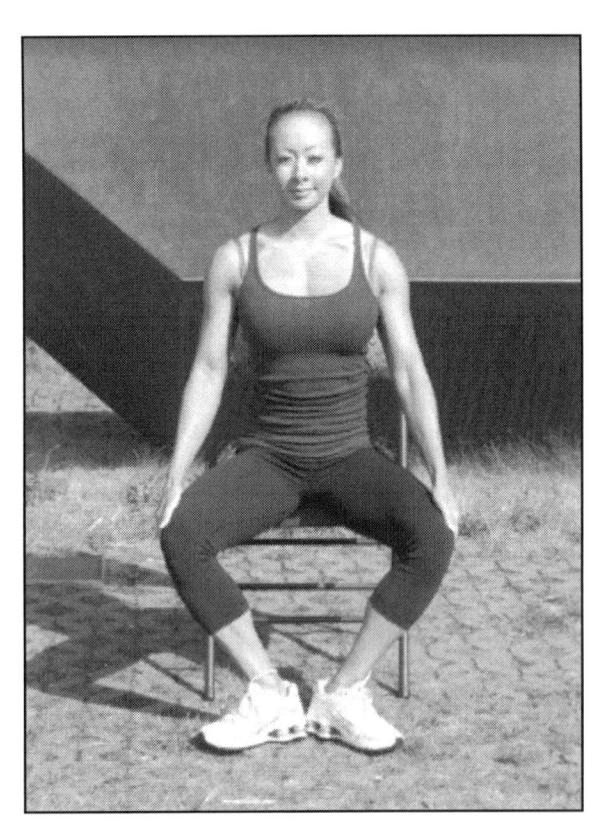

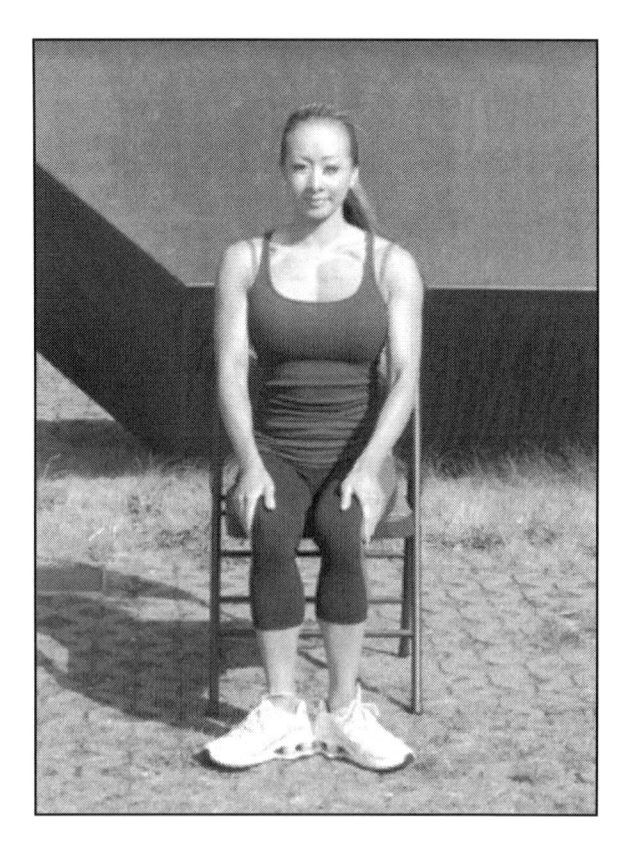

Sitting Leg Flexes

This exercise will develop your inner and outer thighs.

Number Of Repetitions

Beginner: 10 (5 each way) repetitions

Intermediate: 20 (10 each way) repetitions

Advanced: 40 (20 each way) repetitions

How To Perform The Exercise

1. Sit down on the edge of a chair with your feet together and your knees apart.
2. Place the palm of your hands on the inside of your knees.
3. Bring your knees together while offering resistance with your hands and then press your knees apart again.
4. Only offer resistance as you bring your knees together.
5. Once you have completed the required repetitions with your hands on the inside of your knees, repeat this motion with your hands on the outside of your knees. This time, only offer resistance when you separate your knees.

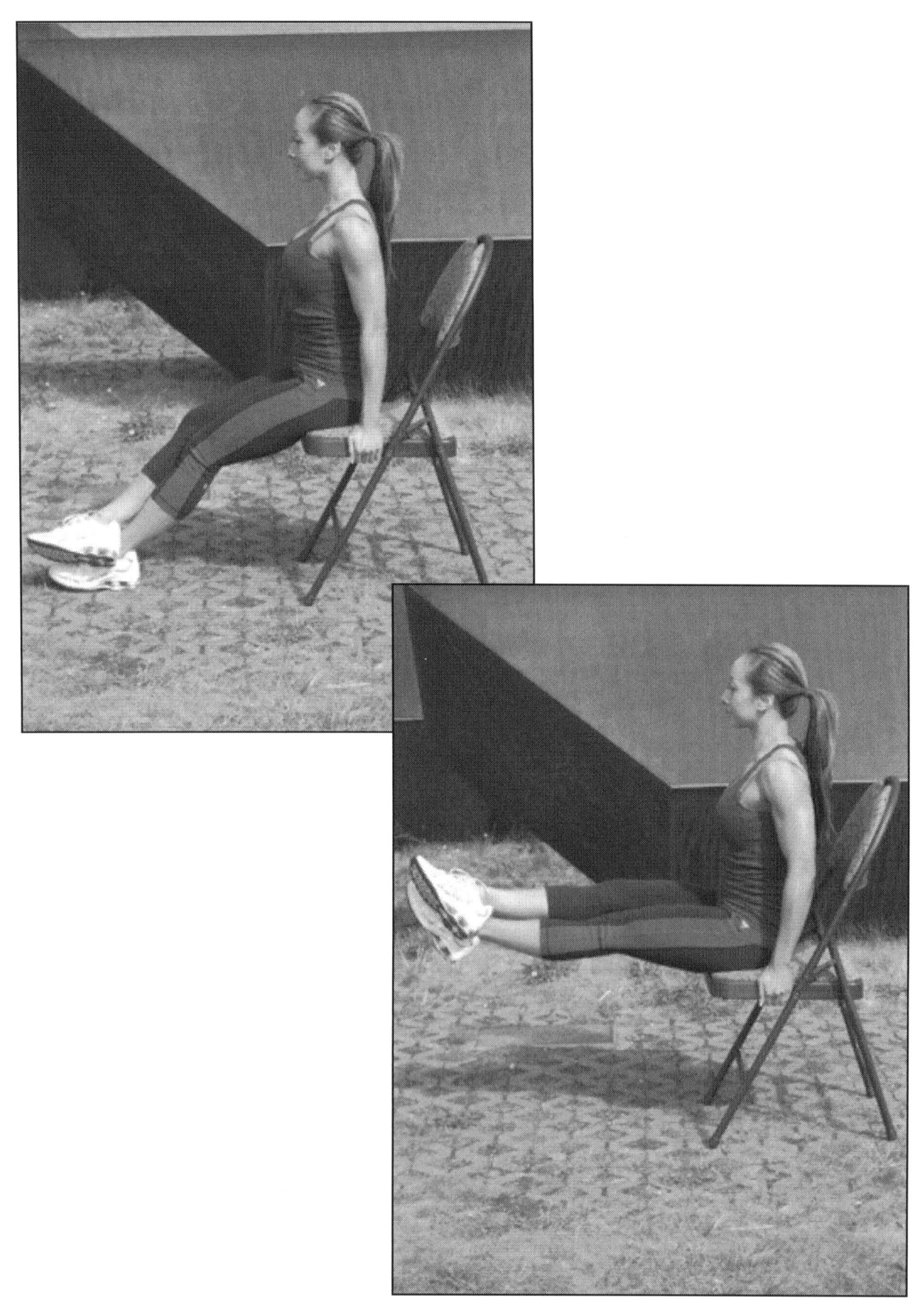

Copyright © 2010 David Nordmark. All rights reserved.
www.animal-kingdom-workouts.com

Page 114

Sitting Leg Extensions

This exercise will develop the front of your thighs.

Number Of Repetitions

Beginner: 10 (5 per leg) repetitions

Intermediate: 20 (10 per leg) repetitions

Advanced: 40 (20 per leg) repetitions

How To Perform The Exercise

1. Sit down in a chair and grab the sides of the seat with your hands for support.
2. Place the heel of your left foot over the instep of your right ankle.
3. Straighten your right leg while providing resistance with your left leg.
4. Perform the required number of repetitions and then switch legs.

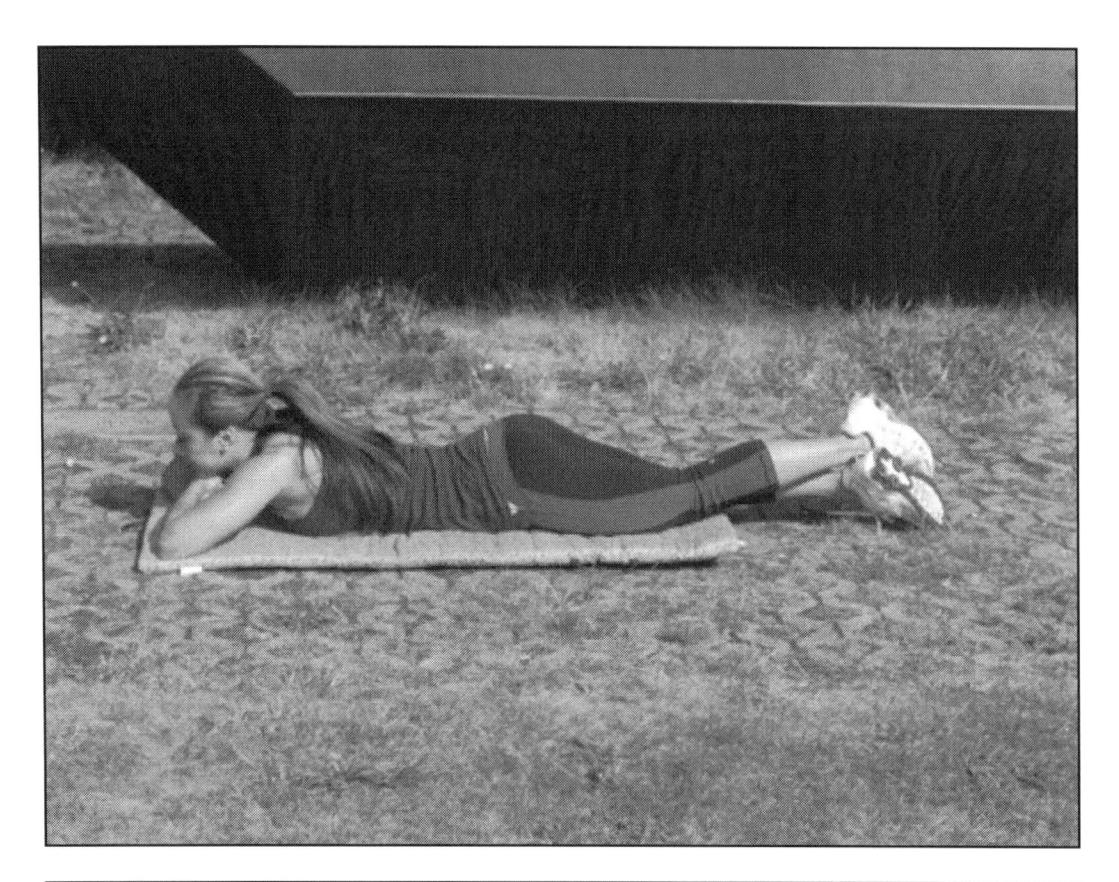

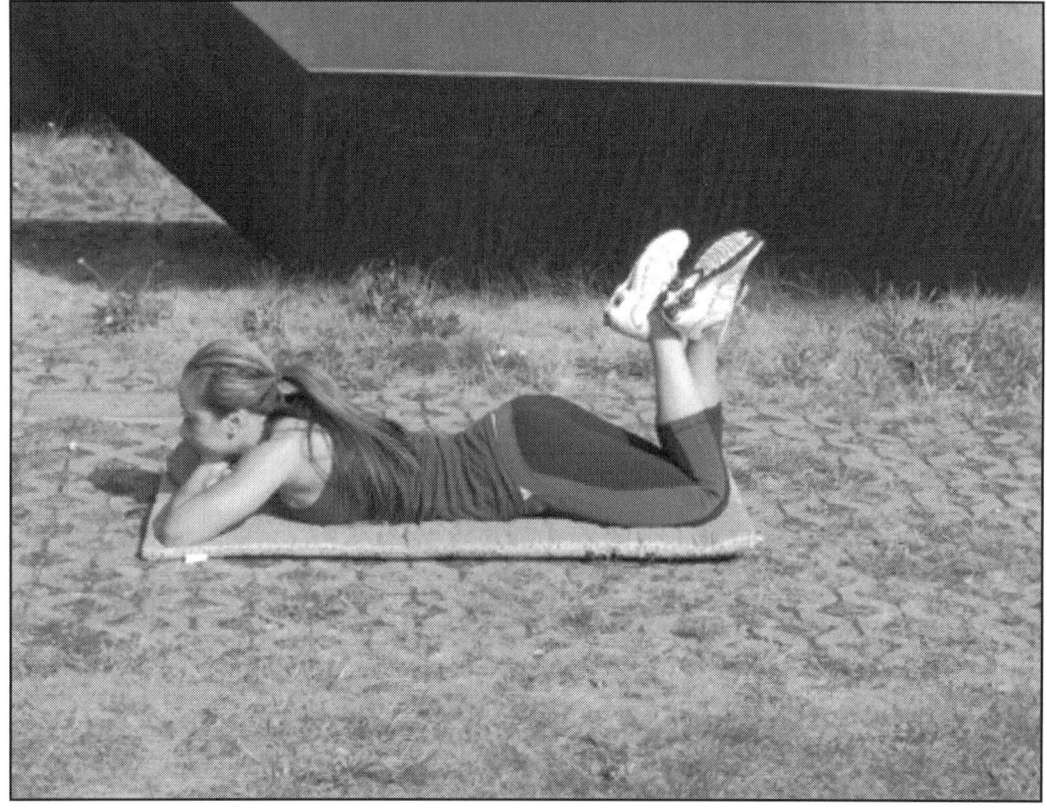

Leg Curls

This exercise will develop your hamstrings.

Number Of Repetitions

Beginner: 10 (5 per leg) repetitions

Intermediate: 20 (10 per leg) repetitions

Advanced: 40 (20 per leg) repetitions

How To Perform The Exercise

1. Lie face down on a soft surface like a mat or carpet with your stomach on the ground.
2. Rest your head on your hands.
3. Place your left foot over your right ankle. This is the starting position.
4. Breathe in through your nose as you bend your right leg from the knee to a 90 degree angle. Provide resistance with your left foot.
5. Lower you legs to the starting position.
6. Perform the required number of repetitions then switch legs.

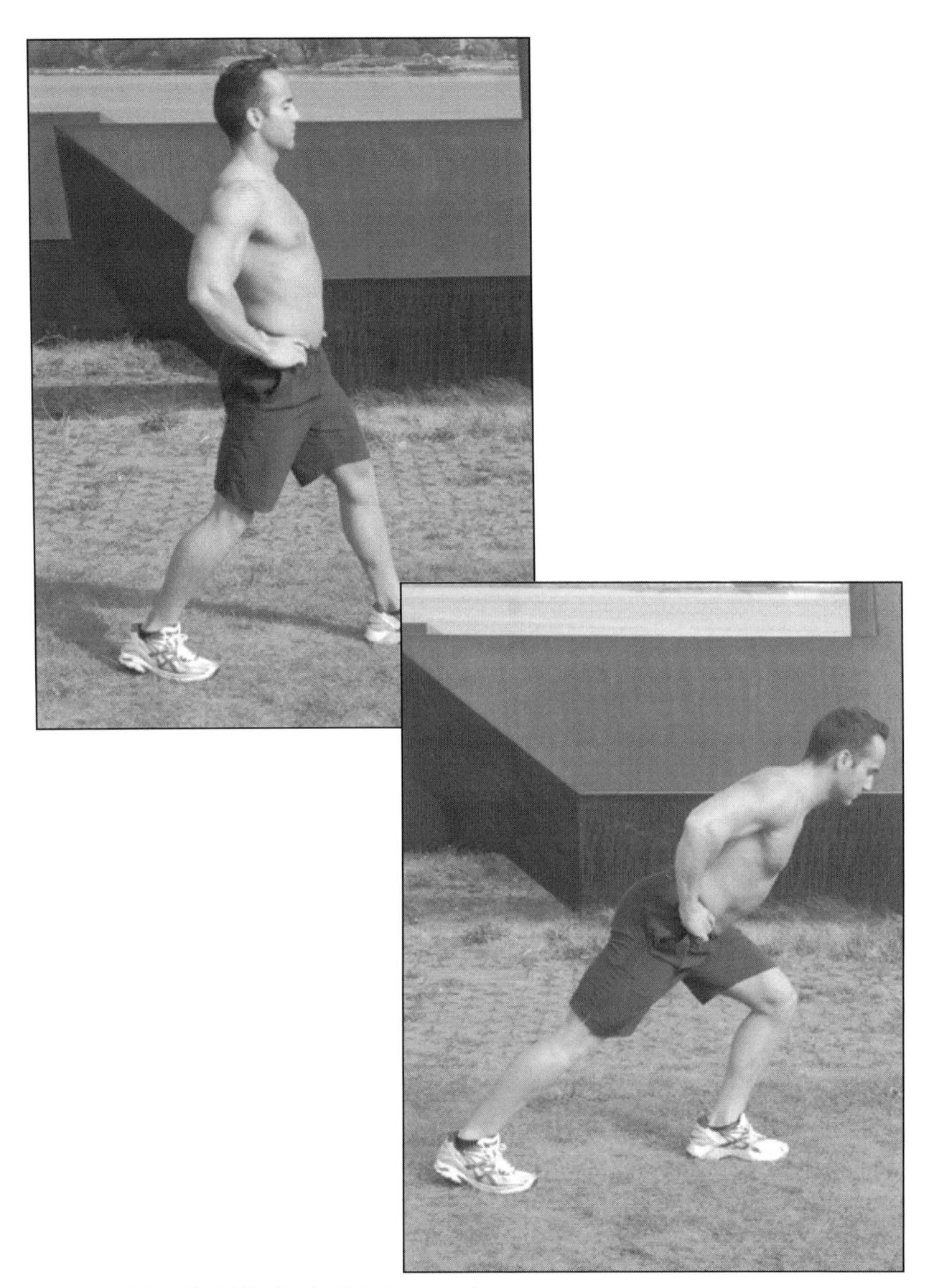

Thigh Flexes

This exercise will develop the muscles in your thighs as well as give your hamstrings a nice stretch.

Number Of Repetitions

Beginner: 10 (5 per leg) repetitions

Intermediate: 20 (10 per leg) repetitions

Advanced: 40 (20 per leg) repetitions

How To Perform The Exercise

1. Begin standing straight up with your right leg forward and your left leg straight behind you.
2. Place your hands on your hips.
3. Bend your right knee so that you lean forward and then press back up again. Keep your left leg straight at all times.
4. Keep you stomach muscles tight and your back straight.
5. Breathe in through your nose as you bend at the knee, breathe out as your press back up.
6. Once you have completed the required repetitions for the right leg switch and work your left leg.

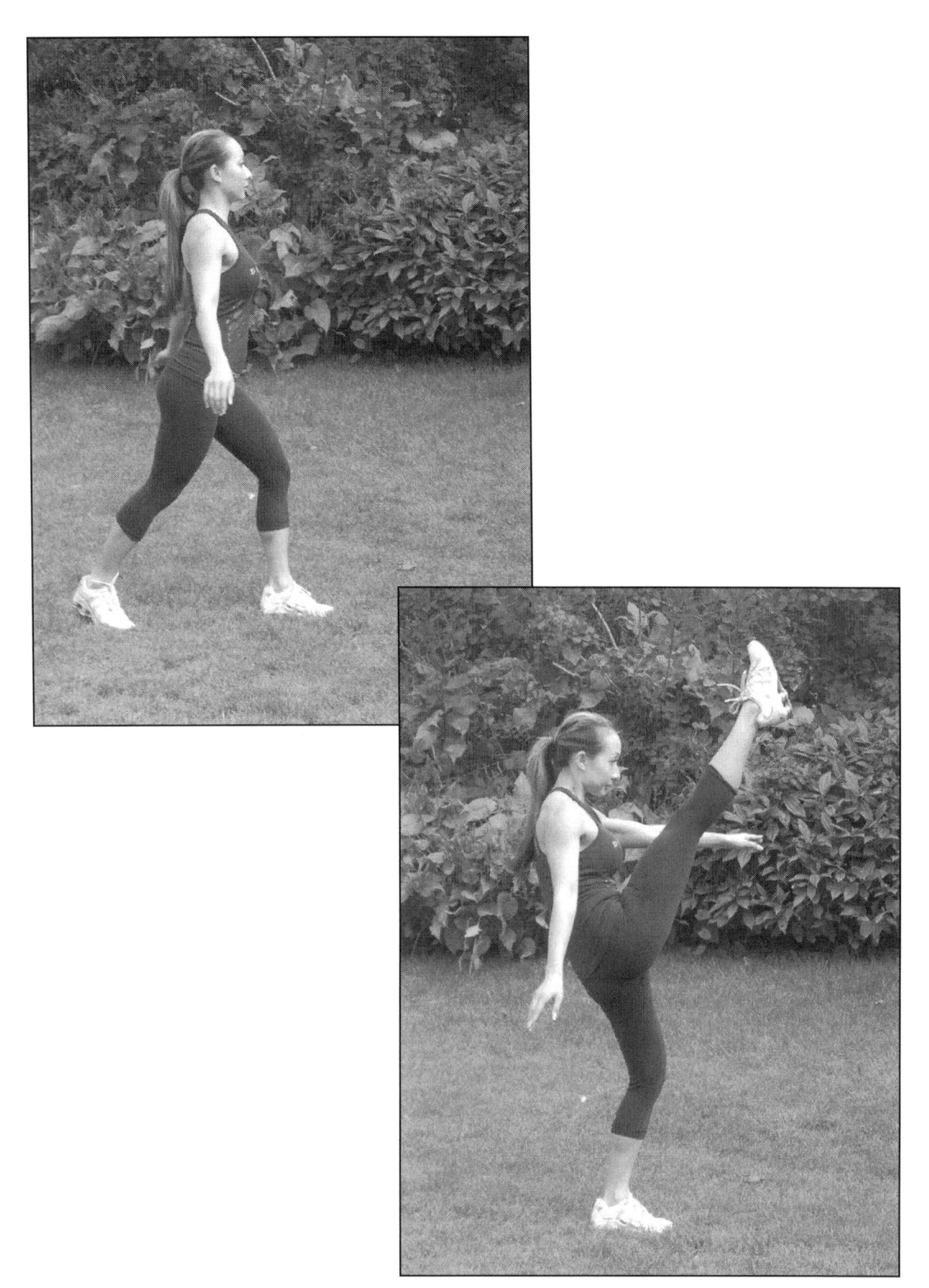

Leg Kicks

This exercise is a three part movement that will strengthen and loosens your hip flexors.

Number Of Repetitions

Beginner: 15 (5 per movement) repetitions

Intermediate: 30 (10 per movement) repetitions

Advanced: 45 (15 per movement) repetitions

How To Perform The Exercise

1. Stand straight up with your right leg behind your left leg.
2. Place your hands on your hips.
3. The first movement is to kick your right leg up 5 times for the beginner level.
4. The second movement is to kick in a circle in fashion. This means to kick the right leg outwards in a circular motion and then to bring it in straight behind you.
5. The third movement involves kicking in a circular out fashion. This means kicking straight out in front of you and then in a circular motion back to the starting position.
6. Once you have completed the required repetitions for the right leg switch and work your left.
7. If you are having a tough time keeping your balance due to the nature of the kicks it is fine to hold onto a chair for balance.

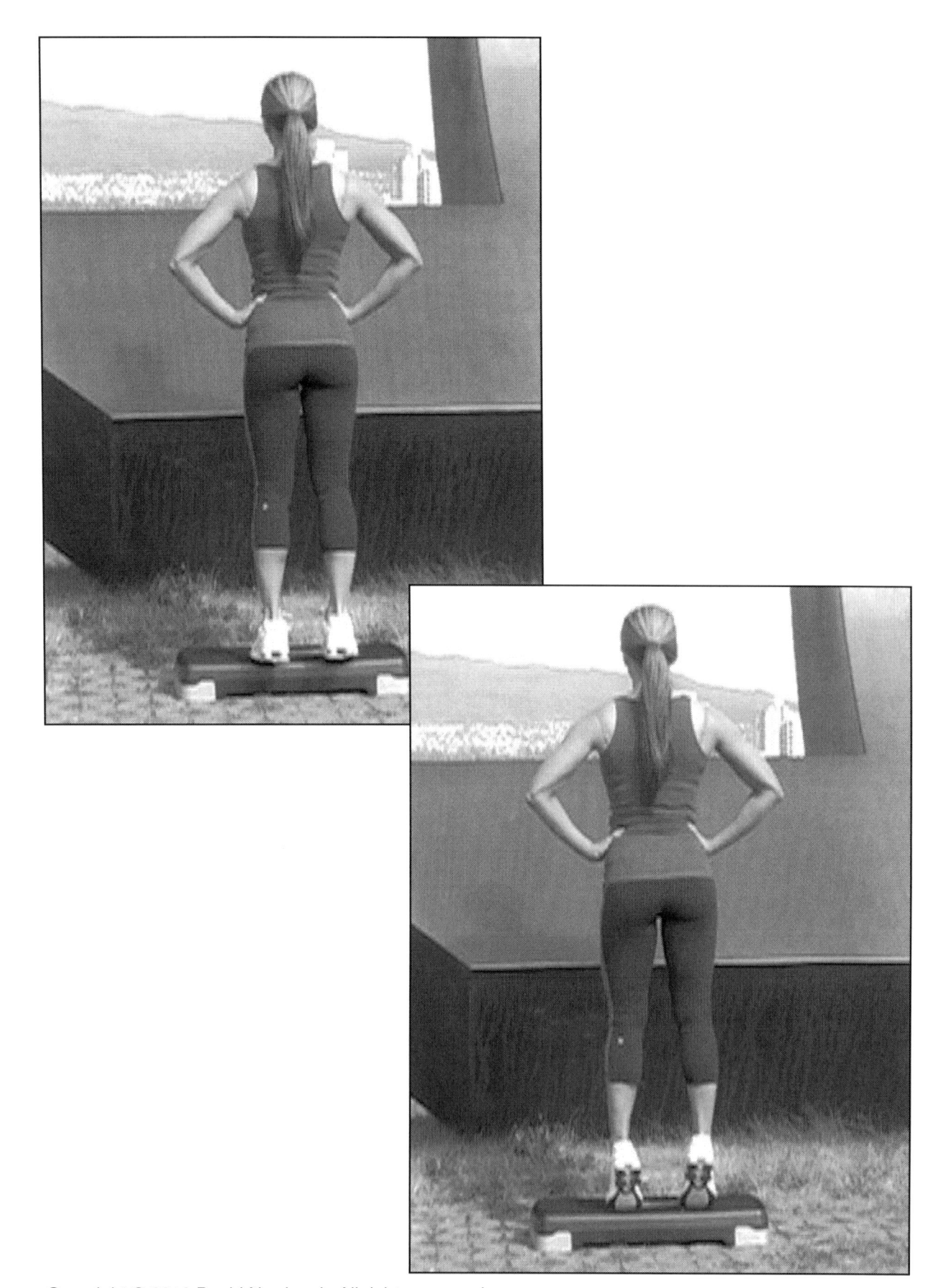

Calve Press Ups

This exercise will develop your calve muscles.

Number Of Repetitions

Beginner: 15 repetitions

Intermediate: 30 repetitions

Advanced: 50 repetitions

How To Perform The Exercise

1. Stand with the balls of your feet on the edge of a stair, thick book, or a block of wood.
2. Lower your heels and then rise up on your toes as high as possible until you feel your calves tense.
3. Lock your calves for a second and then repeat this exercise.
4. Feel free to grab onto a chair or similar object to keep your balance.
5. When you can do 50 or more start doing them one foot at a time.

Other Courses

Natural Fitness - Natural *Bodyweight Exercises* for Men *and* Women (Now Available!)

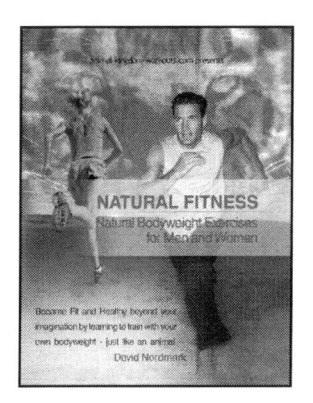

Animals are able to get as strong and healthy as they are by using nothing but their own bodyweight. If you want to be strong and healthy, the kind of person who turns heads, you would be wise to follow their example. In this book I teach you the best bodyweight exercises I know off. They can be done anywhere at anytime, in a little as 15 minutes a day. Take the first steps to a new you today.

To Order The Book - https://www.createspace.com/3453949

Animal Stretching - The Complete Book of Static Stretching, Dynamic Movements, Joint Loosening, Deep Breathing and Energy Exercises

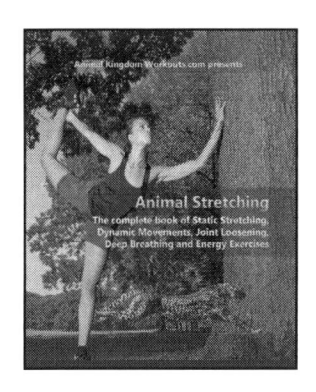

Animal Stretching is more than just another stretching book. Although it does contain its fair share of classic static stretches and routines it also outlines some fantastic deep breathing, joint loosening, dynamic movements and energy exercises that can help you feel fantastic in no time. If you want to increase your flexibility, improve your performance in a sport, get rid of nagging pain or injuries, increase your energy levels or simply feel great again Animal Stretching is for you!

To Order The Book - https://www.createspace.com/3457018

Animal Workouts - Animal-*Inspired* Strength and Conditioning Workouts for *Men* and *Women*

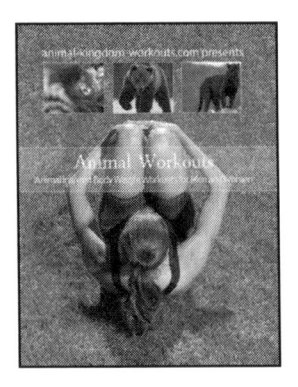

In "*Natural Fitness - Natural Body Weight Exercises for Men and Women*", I outlined some of the best bodyweight exercises I know of to get you in animal-like shape. In this book, I show you (with Karen and Kerry's help!) exercises that are truly based on animal movements. What makes these animal workouts truly unique from anything on the market is how FUN they are. You've probably never seen anything like them. These exercises work great as a complement to "Natural Fitness", or they can be an incredibly effective workout all on their own.

To Order The Book - https://www.createspace.com/3416074

To Order The DVD - https://www.createspace.com/290885

Power Isometrics - The Complete Course that Allows you to Build a Strong an Athletic Body in only 30 Minutes a Day!

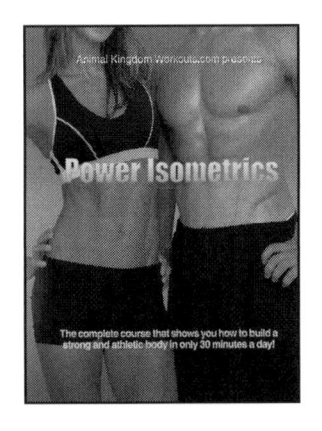

Isometric exercise, which is the science of creating a powerful muscular contraction with no movement, has been around for thousands of years and utilized in such disciplines as Yoga and the Martial Arts. Power Isometrics is a modern take on this time proven discipline that will allow you to build the body of your dreams in less than 1/2 hour a day. Do you want to learn the secret of how to reshape your physique and add strength beyond imagination without ever moving a muscle? Do you want to look and feel your best at all times? Do you want to create lean, perfectly sculpted muscles, shed fat and achieve the glow of perpetual youthfulness without ever having to go to a gym or invest in expensive equipment? Power Isometrics can show you how.

To Order The Book - https://www.createspace.com/3403053

To Order The DVD - https://www.createspace.com/277327

Copyright © 2010 David Nordmark. All rights reserved.
www.animal-kingdom-workouts.com

The Ultimate Guide To Pushups

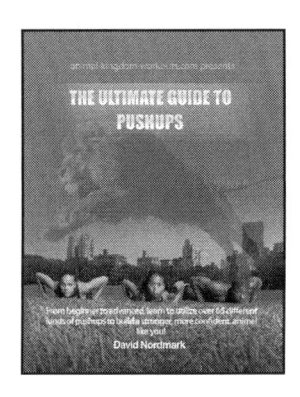

Pushups are one of the oldest and most effective exercises known to man. By themselves pushups work the entire body and can build incredible strength, power, and endurance in record time. The Ultimate Guide To Pushups contains over 65 different pushup variations which are suitable for everyone from the complete beginner to the advanced athlete. You don't need expensive gym memberships or other gimmicks to get in superior shape. The pushup variations presented in this book work most major muscle groups, are free, can be done anywhere at anytime, have a very low chance of injury and, most of all, are fun! If you want to get started on the road to superior natural health then The Ultimate Guide To Pushups is for you!

To Order The Book - https://www.createspace.com/3443359

About the Author

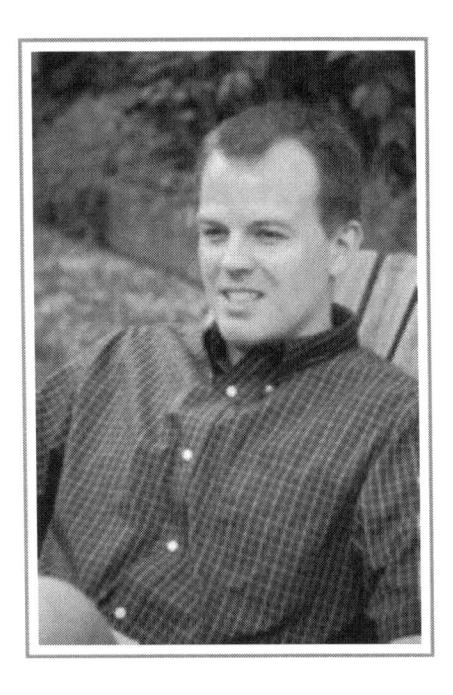

David Nordmark has a life-long interest in health and fitness. In the past he has participated in such sports as soccer, basketball and hockey. He also was once an avid runner and weightlifter but has since come to his senses. Today he mainly does natural exercises like yoga, isometrics and the bodyweight exercises found on his website, www.animal-kingdom-workouts.com. He is also available as a personal fitness trainer to those who are really committed to changing their health and lifestyle for the better. Information on this can be found on his website: www.animal-kingdom-workouts.com

David lives in beautiful Vancouver, British Columbia Canada, although he really wouldn't mind living somewhere else during the winter. He's currently working on making that dream a reality.

If you have any questions for him, feel free to contact him using the contact form that can be found on his website. Here's the link:

http://www.animal-kingdom-workouts.com/contactme.html

About the Models

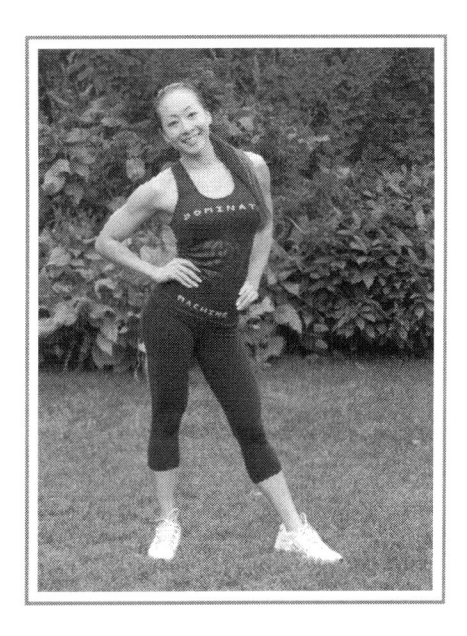

Karen Pang is a Vancouver based fitness model and competitor. She also travels frequently to Los Angeles and Toronto. She is available for fitness modeling, glamour and bikini shoots. She can be reached at karen@misskarenpang.com or through her website at www.misskarenpang.com. To view her portfolio, visit

http://www.modelmayhem.com/558190

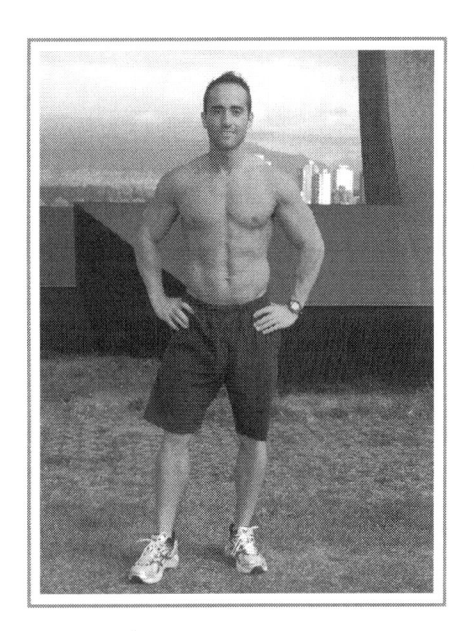

Sean Stewart is a specialized personal fitness trainer and fitness consultant. Sean also does coaching, acting, fitness modeling and online marketing. You may contact him by email at fitmanfrombc@gmail.com or through his website at

www.SeanFitness.com.

Made in the USA
Columbia, SC
04 January 2022